The Carbon Dioxide Syndrome

Learn why changing your breathing can improve your health and wellbeing

Jennifer Stark and Russell Stark

Authors: Jennifer and Russell Stark

Illustrators: Tony Musson and Michael Mostina

© 2002 Buteyko On Line Ltd.
P O Box 81089,
Whenuapai, Auckland,
New Zealand
ISBN 0-473-09610-2

The
Carbon Dioxide
Syndrome

Contents

Important Note

This book is not designed to be a substitute for professional medical and psychological advice, or a guide for self-treatment. It is purely intended as a resource to help you understand how breathing affects the entire body and why the Buteyko Method may be useful if you have health problems that are hyperventilation-related.

Introduction

This book is dedicated to all 'hidden hyperventilators' and is designed to provide an overview of how the Buteyko Institute Method works and why it helps certain illnesses and diseases. It is not a self-help book.

People with asthma, hay fever or panic attacks who want to alleviate their symptoms are constantly on the lookout for information about their condition and why it occurs. While the powers of observation are tested in the search, often only the obvious is noted: 'Cats give me asthma because I inhale their dander.' Teachers of the Buteyko Method, however, have found that a large percentage of the population does not breathe correctly, and in fact breathes more air than is required for everyday living. Once the effects of breathing are examined, this explains why many of these problems occur.

It is difficult to imagine that there is anything wrong with the way you breathe – 'How can I breathe incorrectly? Breathing is so important that if I wasn't doing it properly then I would die, right?' Wrong! Other important functions, such as blood pressure can also become abnormal without you knowing about it and without killing you.

To establish if your breathing has changed, first of all think back to find out if you breathed through your mouth when you were a healthy child. Did your family own cats, yet you did not have asthma? Has snoring only developed since you had that bad cold a few years ago, or since you moved house and perhaps started getting hay fever? Are you less fit now, yet still trying to do as much and go as fast as you did when you were a younger?

The Buteyko Institute Method (BIM) is a series of breathing

exercises and principles of breathing, which provide you with easy ways of discovering your triggers and practical techniques to overcome them. It does not involve other modalities of treatment such as physiotherapy breathing exercises, meditation, religion, hypnotherapy, re-birthing, vitamins, special diets, power of positive thinking or equipment. There is no physical contact with the instructor or anyone else in the class.

When the method is applied correctly, normal blood gas pressures and breathing patterns are restored. The body is able to function more efficiently as metabolism and blood pH stabilise, allowing more oxygen to reach tissues. Until the symptoms that were created by hyperventilation, such as poor sleep, breathlessness, panic, tiredness and cold feet diminish considerably, special exercises are practised and certain principles are followed This provides both good health and a greater sense of wellbeing.

Generally people continue to do what they are already doing unless there is a good reason to change. The Buteyko Institute Method not only provides an extremely good reason to change, but also effective ways to achieve this. The Method is primarily used to address the symptoms of Dysfunctional Breathing, Chronic Hyperventilation Syndrome, 'Hidden Hyperventilation' or the Carbon Dioxide Syndrome as it is called in this book. It may also be used by anyone who wishes to improve his or her health, sports performance and general ability to cope with modern living.

The book has been divided into three sections:

1. Background and theory regarding hyperventilation and the Buteyko Method.

2. Description of some of the conditions that Buteyko is able to reduce or eliminate the symptoms of, and an explanation of why this is.
3. Personal stories from a few who either teach the Method or who use Buteyko for their own health.

Chapter Two provides technical information about breathing and internal respiration. It is not entirely necessary to understand this in order to grasp the basics of the Buteyko Method, so it can be omitted if preferred. However, taking the time to read Chapter Two will provide greater comprehension and so may be worth the effort. It is intended that anyone will be able to start reading at any chapter of interest and still have an understanding of the Buteyko view on that particular topic.

'To have a better night's sleep, to wake more rested, to have more energy, to be more hopeful of the future, and to be in control of my asthma, this is what the Buteyko technique has done for me.' Jenny

Jenny's comment and others like it are found throughout the book. They have been taken from survey forms completed by people who attended Buteyko courses taught by Russell or Jennifer Stark.

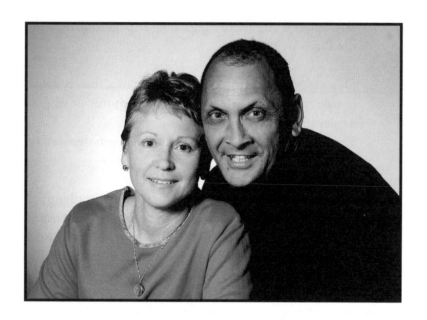

Jennifer and Russell Stark have been teaching the Buteyko Method for more than ten years. Russian practitioner, Alexander Stalmatski trained them in Australia to teach the Method not long before they moved to New Zealand to begin teaching 'Buteyko' there. The Starks not only teach the Buteyko Method but also train other practitioners. They have worked constantly towards having the Buteyko Method recognised in the western world. They became interested in Buteyko primarily for their son who had severe asthma. Russell also had chronic asthma and tells their story:

'My asthma and that of our son Robert had been deteriorating for years when my wife Jen heard about Buteyko. She simply said one night, "I have enrolled you two in a Buteyko course!" and then proceeded to sell the idea to us. She hardly knew anything about it but was convinced that it sounded like a good idea. I was really sceptical and not at all keen to go along the first night, but decided that anything was worth a try because asthma was completely controlling our lives.

Robert was taking at least three nebulisers of Ventolin every day plus an inhaled reliever, inhaled steroid and also Prednisone every few weeks. I was taking puffers all day, every day. Whereas Robert was totally wired by all that adrenaline-type medication charging through his system, I was chronically tired. I had catnaps every day plus going to bed for hours every night. I say "going to bed", because while I lay down for a long time, I seemed to be awake half the time, either needing a drink, going to the bathroom or taking my reliever. In the morning I just wanted to start all over again instead of going to work.

Both of us found the first twenty-four hours of using Buteyko absolutely amazing. Robert didn't use any reliever medication and I only needed it once. It was so amazing that I thought we must have been hypnotised at the class. (At the time, I was half convinced that asthma was a mental condition rather than a physical one.) But as time went on and we got better at overcoming the symptoms as well as the symptom frequency dropping dramatically, I started to think that there had to be something in this "Russian breathing thing".

A few months later when Buteyko Australia asked if I was interested in training, I couldn't wait to start. Now I had the job of convincing Jen that it was a good idea. We were conventional kind of people – normally did exactly what the doctor ordered and so it was really thinking outside the square for us to become involved in a "natural" therapy. I had to almost drag Jen to the training, but she soon became as keen as I was. We decided to take Buteyko to New Zealand because no one was teaching it there, and with New Zealand having the highest rate of asthma in the world, where better to take an asthma treatment? We had no idea of what we were up against.

In New Zealand, the Buteyko Method did not have the media support that it had in Australia, so it was really difficult to introduce something as revolutionary there. Buteyko not only enables people to overcome asthma symptoms, but it also stops people from getting them. This is the hard part for asthmatics to come to grips with. Normally the only way you can have fewer symptoms is by taking more steroids, yet we were saying that most people could cut down or eliminate steroids as well. People looked at us as if we were mad. When most people try to give up their preventers they have a relapse in their condition, so they become convinced that it is impossible.

However, we hung in there and I am really glad of this because we have been able to help thousands of people restore normality to their lives. Having asthma does not just mean a cough, chest tightness or wheezing, it can mean poor sleep patterns, being irritable, having sore muscles and feeling tired all the time. It can completely take over your life. Being without it is an absolutely magic feeling and I am glad that I have played a part in creating an awareness of Buteyko.'

Acknowledgments

Many people have helped us prepare this book and we would like to thank them all for their never-ending patience and good humour.

We give special thanks to both Professor Konstantin Pavlovich Buteyko and our son Robert. Professor Buteyko created the idea and the techniques that have changed our lives forever. These techniques brought our son's debilitating asthma to an abrupt halt. In our desire to help Robert, we learned to teach the Buteyko Institute Method, which has allowed us to help thousands of others. Robert has also contributed to this by creating our web site www.buteyko.co.nz

Chapter 1

How Good is Today's Lifestyle?

The affluence and technology of the developed world has provided clean water, good food, warmth, education and advanced medicine, which could be expected to support excellent health, yet it does not always achieve this.

Today there are health conditions such as asthma, allergies, sleep apnoea, heart disease, hypertension, diabetes, chronic fatigue syndrome, obesity, depression, anxiety and panic attacks in far greater numbers than ever before. For example, by the mid 1990s in Britain the incidence of asthma was double that of the early 1980s, and represented more than 10% of British children (Ridgeway 1994). Figures are comparable in all English-speaking countries. Modern medicine has no cure for asthma or these other conditions because it does not understand or treat the cause. The best that can be offered is medication to reduce some of the symptoms.

Why is This?

One explanation is our increasingly sedentary lifestyle. How healthy would a dog be if it ate six times a day yet seldom went for a walk? How happy would a child be sitting at a desk all day? These things, which have become daily occurrences for many people in the western world, are totally different to the lifestyle of their ancestors. It appears that physically people have changed little for centuries, if skeletons that are found of early humans are at least 40,000 years old, as claimed by scientists. This means that the prototype of the human body in use today is designed to cope best with life, not for today's lifestyle but for one that meant moving around for most of the day, eating a variety of foods when they were available, and going hungry every now and then. It is difficult to imagine how life was in those days so take a look at the lifestyle of just fifty years ago:

In those days housework was mostly done manually with few automatic tools to help out, and over 80% of all employment involved some sort of physical labour. Children spent hours outdoors, walking, running, playing; they helped out on the farm or did chores around the house; there were no videos or computers and few television programmes designed to keep their interest and have them sitting still for hours at a time. In short, life was a lot more physical for everyone. In addition to more physical activity, many foods were not available all year round. Refrigerators were small and inefficient, and the average family did not own a freezer, which meant that most foods were bought fresh, in season and virtually on a daily basis. There were few packaged meals and more emphasis was placed on quantity, rather than taste or appearance. It is not that having fewer choices of food, or working long hours of physical labour is good for everyone, but it better suits the basic human design. Even today, small children, who have yet to learn what is expected of them, respond to their bodily urges. If given the chance, they eat when they are hungry, sleep when they are tired and play in between.

Today most people in developed countries eat at least three times a day - *every* day, whether hungry or not; walking for many is almost a thing of the past apart from the house to the car and parking as close to the destination as possible; hours are spent sitting on the couch watching television, and the days are largely governed by the clock rather than the season. Because this lifestyle does not suit the basic human make-up, it creates stress.

Stress

When the word 'stress' is considered, most people think along the same lines as this explanation from the Reader's Digest dictionary:

> '6.a. A mentally or emotionally disruptive or disquieting influence. b. A state of tension or distress caused by such an influence.'

A more accurate definition of what stress does to the body can be found in medical dictionaries. Dorland (1982) defines stress as:

> 'The sum of the biological reactions to any adverse stimulus, physical, mental, or emotional, internal or external, that tends to disturb an organism's homoeostasis; should compensating reactions be inadequate or inappropriate, stress may lead to various disorders. The term is also used to refer to the stimuli that elicit the reactions.'

Stress expert Dr. Hans Selye (1984) uses another definition when documenting the physical implications of stress. He refers to stress as 'the rate of wear and tear in the body'. Stress keeps your heartbeat high, makes you bite your lip and alters the process that keeps your body functioning properly in a healthy state.

There are many types of stimuli that cause stress, including physical activities, money worries, environment, illness, injury, emotions and family or work-related activities. For example, stress can be generated by exposure to extremes of cold or heat, running up a hill, worrying about the bank balance, being excited about a first date, having an allergy or an infection, laughing hysterically and a myriad of other things. These things create stress throughout the day and when environmental pollutants, overeating and lack of exercise are added, a situation where stress is low-grade but chronic can quickly develop.

When people are exposed to stress they kick start the 'fight or flight' response. Adrenaline surges through the body, increasing heart and breathing rates to enable sudden physical exertion (Perera 1988). This would be perfect if you were Fred Flintstone running from a dinosaur or lifting a boulder, but dinosaur-type stress is very rare today; driving in peak hour traffic, being late and making work deadlines are more common. These kinds of stress require little or no physical action, so revving up the body at these times is of little benefit and may be detrimental in the long term.

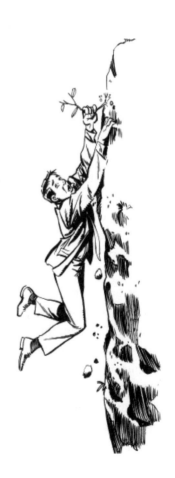

The 'Fight or Flight' Response

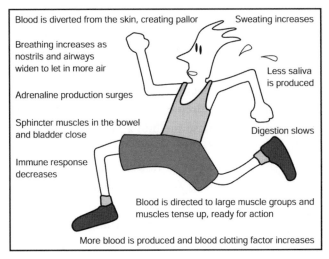

Blood is diverted from the skin, creating pallor

Sweating increases

Breathing increases as nostrils and airways widen to let in more air

Less saliva is produced

Adrenaline production surges

Sphincter muscles in the bowel and bladder close

Digestion slows

Immune response decreases

Blood is directed to large muscle groups and muscles tense up, ready for action

More blood is produced and blood clotting factor increases

Figure 1:1 The 'fight or flight' response is the normal reaction to any dangerous or stressful situation.

As can be seen from Figure 1.1 multiple things happen to keep people safe from danger. For example: adrenaline facilitates fast movement and quick reaction; blood is diverted away from the skin and thickens to lessen potential bleeding; bodily functions such as digestion, which are not required to save oneself, switch off. This enables maximum blood supply and energy to reach large muscle groups. The part of the brain that controls this response is primitive and involuntary and much of it is reflexive. For example, without conscious thought the hand is immediately snatched out of water that is too hot for comfort, or the person freezes at the sound of a growling dog.

For early humans, the fight or flight response was vital for survival because they needed to run from wild animals and hunt for food. Today, the stress is more likely to be caused by taking a flight in an aeroplane. Perhaps it is the fear of flying, the sadness of in the plane, or the lack of physical movement for a number of hours.

The fight or flight response can be activated by other events normally considered safe or fun, such as becoming caught up in the drama of an action movie. While watching the hero walk into a trap, the person becomes mildly anxious on his behalf and the primitive brain prepares for action by triggering the necessary responses. These include a faster breathing pattern, dry mouth, extra energy and increased heartbeat. After a short time, the physical difference is noticed and while one person might decide to get a drink of water, another might become aware of how hot they feel and start to worry. Worry only makes the response stronger, with even faster breathing and heart rate. In this situation the fight or flight response is activated unnecessarily and might provoke extra stress.

It doesn't matter what creates the stress, the fact remains that if it cannot be fought or avoided, and it is either long term or repeated frequently, the natural response may be detrimental to the person's health. For example, the release of the extra blood clotting factor may cause deep vein thrombosis in a susceptible person. In this instance, the natural fight or flight response to stress will have actually created a problem instead of providing a solution.

General Adaptation Syndrome

Selye explains that when faced with any stress, the body can only respond in two ways: (1) advance and fight it or (2) ignore it or run away. In either case, he calls the first stage of the response the 'Alarm Reaction', the second is the 'Stage of Resistance' and the third, the 'Stage of Exhaustion'. These make up the General

Adaptation Syndrome, which takes over when the homoeostatic mechanisms cannot maintain the usual internal environment (Bradley 2000, Tortora 1984). Under normal circumstances, homoeostasis deals with everyday stresses such as walking into a hot room, by automatically causing extra perspiration so that the internal temperature stays the same. If the normal temperature cannot be maintained then the General Adaptation Syndrome is activated, and while superficially the person appears well, their internal environment is not normal. For example, blood pressure and sugar levels will be higher than usual while coping with the stress of being too hot.

The General Adaptation Syndrome can be demonstrated by imagining a man walking down the road when a savage dog runs out onto the footpath. The fight or flight response switches on, but he gets bitten on the leg before managing to escape. Since the man cannot run from the injury, he must fight it and so the Alarm Reaction continues with a huge response as the whole body reacts with intensified heartbeat, breathing and blood flow that bring histamine and other chemicals to the area. After the initial 'Alarm Reaction', the rest of the man's body calms down but his leg is still greatly affected. Heat, swelling and pains are felt as the immune system fights to keep the infection in one place, which is the Stage of Resistance. If the immune system cannot contain or kill the infection it will spread further into his body and once again the whole body becomes involved. If the situation was extreme and the effort to fight the infection was too great, the 'Stage of Exhaustion' would be reached and the man would die. But of course most stress reactions are minor and only those of an extreme nature result in death.

Of all the responses to stress, perhaps the one least likely to be noticed is the increase in breathing. Despite breathing having a profound effect on the entire body, it is seldom checked to see if it is normal. An abnormal breathing pattern, or 'dysfunctional breathing', creates an imbalance of the gases found in the bloodstream, which in turn leads to an overall downturn in health, as well as a greater susceptibility to further stress. Stress is not necessarily a bad thing, and the only person who does not have any stress is already dead. However, when stress is prolonged or the reaction to the stress is not channelled correctly, it can cause health problems (Fried 1993).

References

Bradley D. Hyperventilation Syndrome. Tandem Press. Auckland. 2000. pp427-428

Dorland. Dorland's Pocket Medical Dictionary. Philadelphia: W.B. Saunders Company. 1982

Fried R. The Psychology and Physiology of Breathing. Plenum Press. New York 1993. p217

Perera, J. The Hazards of Heavy Breathing. New Scientist. 1988. Dec. pp. 46-48

Ridgeway, R. Asthma. Shaftesbury, UK: Element Books Ltd. 1994. Introduction.

Selye, H. The Stress of Life. New York: McGraw-Hill. 1984. Preface xvi & pp. 111-127

Tortora GJ, Anagnostakos NP. Principles of Anatomy and Physiology. Harper & Row, New York. 1984. p560

Chapter 2

Breathing: the Most Basic Need

The Buteyko Method is about restoring normal breathing patterns in spite of the continued stress of today's lifestyle, so that the symptoms caused by dysfunctional breathing are eliminated or greatly diminished and good health becomes more likely. The next few pages describe the workings of the respiratory system. It is not essential to fully comprehend this information, but taking the time to read it will give you a greater understanding of breathing and breathing - related health problems. If you prefer to get started on more hands-on information then turn to Chapter 3.

Breathing is an automatic process like the heart beating, and it occurs at least 20,000 times a day. To a certain extent it is possible to alter the speed and depth of breathing simply by deciding to, such as when speaking, which is contrary to the control of most automatic processes. For example, it is not possible to voluntarily speed up or stop digestion or hair growth. Because this limited control over breathing is available, it is possible to deliberately make changes to the pattern for short periods of time, which will begin to change the automatic programming the rest of the time.

The main purpose of breathing is to supply the body with sufficient oxygen, to remove excess carbon dioxide and to maintain a constant pH in the bloodstream (Naifeh 1994). The breathing is automatically adjusted as necessary to meet these demands. Healthy people use only their nose and diaphragm to breathe with when sleeping, sitting or walking, but during exercise, when oxygen requirements are greater and the body produces more carbon dioxide, breathing speeds up and larger breaths are taken. If the exercise is particularly strenuous, the mouth and strong upper chest muscles are used temporarily to move lots of air in and out of the lungs, but on returning to a state of rest, nose breathing and sole use of the diaphragm starts again.

Sometimes this automatic adjustment becomes dysfunctional, and if breathing is deeper or faster than is required to supply sufficient oxygen and to remove excess carbon dioxide, it is called 'hyperventilation'. Breathing through the mouth or using the upper chest muscles when you are resting may not seem excessive, but it causes an imbalance of the blood gases and pH, which is detrimental in the long term.

Survival and Carbon Dioxide

There are three things that are needed in order for people to survive: food, water and oxygen. People can go several weeks without food, a few days without water, but only minutes without oxygen, making breathing the most important of these survival requirements.

Oxygen acts like a fuel, combining with pyruvic acid (a breakdown of glucose) within the tissue cells to provide people with energy to stay alive and to function, or in other words to meet the demands of metabolism. Metabolism is the amount of energy, or the sum of all the chemical processes and physical reactions it takes to stay alive and run, walk or sleep.

Often carbon dioxide is considered to be unimportant or simply a waste gas because it is the end result of this process, along with energy and water. In fact carbon dioxide is the regulator of all bodily functions either directly or indirectly, making it the fourth requirement of survival. Without it, death would occur (Anderson Price 1992). Yandell Henderson was an American scientist who did much study on breathing and carbon dioxide in the early part of the twentieth century. He is quoted here from the 1940 edition of Cyclopedia of Medicine:

'Modern physiology has shown that, in addition to the control and regulation exerted by the nervous system, there are many chemical substances produced in the body that influence function and form. To these active principles Starling gave the name of "hormones." Among the hormones are epinephrine (often called adrenaline), pituitrin, thyroxin, insulin and many other products of the glands of internal secretion and other organs.

Carbon dioxide is the chief hormone of the entire body; it is the only one that is produced by every tissue and that probably acts on every organ. In the regulation of the functions of the body, carbon dioxide exerts at least 3 well-defined influences: (1) It is one of the prime factors in the acid-base balance of the blood. (2) It is the principal control of respiration. (3) It exerts an essential tonic influence upon the heart and peripheral circulation.'

Professor Konstantin Pavlovich Buteyko, founder of the Buteyko Method, also had strong views on the importance of carbon dioxide, as is revealed in this interview circa 1980:

'The theory of life, in brief, is such that carbon dioxide is the basic nutrition of every life form on Earth – if it disappears, there will be no life on Earth. It acts as the regulator of all functions in the organism; it maintains the internal environment of the organism; it is the vitamin of all vitamins.'

The most important functions that carbon dioxide is involved with are:

- Regulation of the breathing pattern
- Control of blood flow to the brain and to the body's extremities
- Haemoglobin and oxygen affinity
- Maintenance of pH of bodily fluids
- Regulation of pH inside nerve cells
- Facilitation of message-sending by nerves
- Control of the balance between the sympathetic and parasympathetic nervous systems (Lum 1978).

A Balance is Needed

If breathing is not kept at the level necessary to meet the demands of metabolism, the stores of carbon dioxide and oxygen that are kept in the body become unbalanced. This causes a problem because these gases rely on each other to keep the body performing at the highest possible standard. Having sufficient oxygen but insufficient carbon dioxide does not provide this high standard, and neither does the reverse.

While having insufficient carbon dioxide or oxygen can be fatal, so too can excessive amounts of both gases. Antioxidants help to deal with too much oxygen in the form of 'free radicals', and the volume of oxygen entering the bloodstream is normally limited by lung design and haemoglobin content. An excess of carbon dioxide is usually avoided because it is constantly being removed when exhaling. The constant aim, therefore, is to have the optimum balance of both carbon dioxide and oxygen to ensure good health.

pH

The various pH values within the body are factors that also require a careful balance, because having the correct pH is essential for all living organisms. The pH of a substance is the measure of acidity or alkalinity within that substance, and is calculated by the concentration of hydrogen ions on a scale of zero to fourteen. When the concentration of hydrogen ions is high, the pH is acidic and the pH number is less than seven. When the concentration is low, the substance is alkaline and the pH number is above seven.

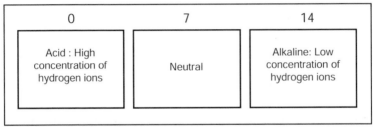

Figure 2:1. The pH scale.

The pH values of fluids found in the body differ from each other. For example digestive juice produced by the stomach is acidic, with a normal value of between 1.2 and 3.0. Bile however, which is also used in digestion, is alkaline and has a pH range from 7.6 to 8.6. In the arterial blood the pH is alkaline and ranges between 7.35 and 7.45, with 7.4 being the norm (Tortora 1984).

Breathing and the pH of arterial blood are reliant on each other to a large extent because breathing plays an important role in regulating the pH of the blood, and the pH of the blood reciprocates by regulating the breathing. If the pH of the blood alters due to abnormal breathing patterns, the person is said to have either 'Respiratory Acidosis' or 'Respiratory Alkalosis'

(Guyton 1982). For example, if a person's arterial blood has a pH of 7.3 due to their breathing, then it would be said that the person is in a state of 'Respiratory Acidosis'; if the pH was 7.5 then it would be 'Respiratory Alkalosis'. The pH can also change due to metabolic disturbances that have nothing to do with breathing. For example, 'Metabolic Acidosis' can be caused by having diarrhoea and 'Metabolic Alkalosis' can be caused by excessive vomiting (Tortora 1984).

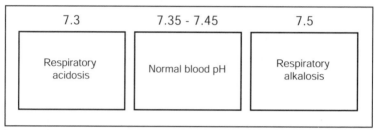

Figure 2:2. The blood pH range is narrow.

Even quite small changes to the pH of the bloodstream are dangerous to life. So while it is perfectly acceptable to have the saliva pH at 6.5, if the blood were at this point the person would be dead because blood pH extremes of 6.8 or 7.8 for any length of time will cause death. The brain, therefore, strives to keep the pH within the healthy range (Anderson Price 1992, Guyton 1982).

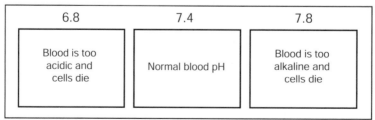

Figure 2:3. Sudden changes or changes to the pH that are too great can kill.

However, the brain will adapt to a different pH providing this change is small. This is of benefit when relaxing and preparing for sleep because the pH of the blood decreases marginally, anaesthetising the nervous system and allowing sleep. In the morning, the daytime breathing pattern resumes to restore usual waking pH, which stimulates the nervous system into its usual activity (Piper 1992). People who live at high altitude have chronic Respiratory Alkalosis and some people with emphysema have the opposite (Guyton 1982, Lumb 2000). Both groups of people slowly develop an abnormal blood pH and in spite of impaired health, they can remain in these states for years. Because small changes can be made to the pH, the Buteyko Method techniques are able to restore a normal breathing pattern.

Gas Laws: Exchange of Pressure and the Effect on Breathing

- Gases exert pressure or tension and this pressure is measured in mm Hg (millimetres of mercury). This means that the pressure is sufficient to support a column of mercury of that height. For example, 40 mm Hg means that the pressure of the gas will hold up a column of mercury that is 40 millimetres high.
- When gas is put into two jars of the same size, the jar with the most gas has the highest pressure. When the same amount of gas is put into both a large jar and a small jar, the pressure of the gas in the small jar will be higher. (Boyle's Law).
- When more than one gas is mixed together, each gas has its own *partial pressure* of the total pressure. According to Dalton's Law, each gas exerts the same pressure when it is mixed with other gases, as if it were the only gas in the volume.

- Gases always try to equalise their own partial pressure or tension regardless of the presence of other gases. They move from areas where the pressure is high to a connected area where it is low. The atmosphere, lungs, blood and tissues are like a series of interconnected jars, and gases constantly move between them to equalise their own partial pressure.

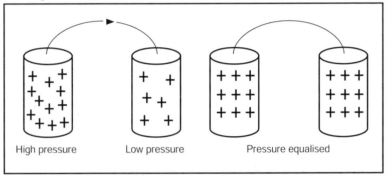

High pressure   Low pressure   Pressure equalised

Figure 2:4. When two jars are connected, gases move between the two jars until their own partial pressure is equal.

- Atmospheric pressure is the sum of all the gas tensions in the atmosphere. Due to gravity atmospheric pressure at sea level is higher than at altitude. When atmospheric pressure is discussed it usually refers to the sea level pressure (760 mm Hg). The sum of the partial pressures of gases inside the body has to be virtually the same as atmospheric pressure – otherwise the body would explode or be crushed.

- Approximately 21% of atmospheric air is oxygen but it contains virtually no carbon dioxide, so while oxygen is obtained from the atmosphere, carbon dioxide is synthesized by metabolism. Any loss or retention relies on breathing. When the breath is held carbon dioxide pressure increases, and when more is breathed out than is being produced, the pressure drops.

Respiration

Respiration literally means to 're-breathe', and is controlled by the 'respiratory centre', which is a group of nerves found in the brain stem. It is estimated that when a healthy person is resting, between four and six litres of air is moved in and out of the body each minute. This occurs in the average ten - fourteen breaths taken, with each approximately somewhat less than half a litre, perhaps 350 mil of air (Guyton 1982).

There are five parts to the breathing process:

1. The movement of air in and out of the lungs
2. The exchange of oxygen and carbon dioxide between the lungs and the blood
3. Carrying these gases around the body in the bloodstream
4. The exchange of oxygen and carbon dioxide between the blood and the tissues
5. The use of oxygen by the tissues and the production of carbon dioxide.

Air Movement in the Lungs

Air travels through the nose and mouth, down the throat and into the lungs, through what is known as the 'bronchial tree'. This is a series of breathing tubes or airways that become progressively smaller and lead into tiny air sacs called alveoli, which is where the blood absorbs oxygen and releases excess carbon dioxide. The rest of the air remains in what is called the 'dead air space', which includes the nose, throat and large upper airways where gas exchange does not take place.

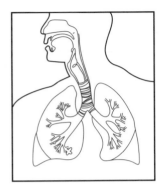
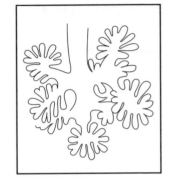

Figure 2:5. The Bronchial tree.   *Figure 2:6. Alveoli.*

Because the lungs are comprised of ever-narrowing tubes, they always retain some air inside them. Only approximately one seventh of the newly inhaled air reaches the alveoli (Guyton 1982), ensuring that the gas mix in the alveoli is totally different to that of the atmosphere. For example, oxygen represents 21% of atmospheric air but only 14% of the alveolar air, and carbon dioxide is almost nonexistent in the atmosphere at 0.04%, yet takes up approximately 6% of the air in the alveoli. If the lungs were not designed in this way, oxygen pressure in the bloodstream would be too high and carbon dioxide pressure too low, causing death.

Airways are composed of three layers – an outer muscular sheath, an inner lining and on the inside are tiny hair-like cilia that move a blanket of mucus, protecting and cleaning the airways. The outer layer is wrapped in 'smooth' or involuntary muscle, which unlike skeletal muscle cannot be consciously moved.

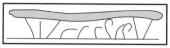

Figure 2:7. Cilia and the mucus blanket.

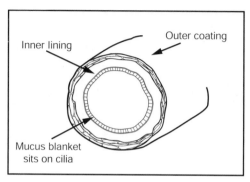

Figure 2:8. Healthy airway.

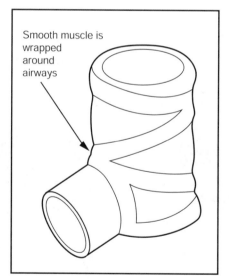

Figure 2:9. Airway Smooth Muscle.

When inhaling, the diaphragm contracts and lowers, the chest and lungs expand, dropping air pressure in the lungs to below atmospheric pressure. Following the principles of Boyle's Law, air rushes into the lungs until the pressure has equalised.

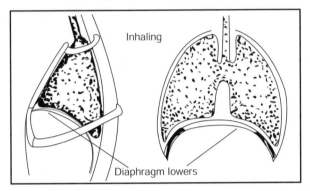

Figure 2:10. The diaphragm contracts and lowers in order to suck air into the lungs.

On exhalation, the diaphragm relaxes, shrinking lung space and raising air pressure to above atmospheric pressure. Now air flows out until the tensions are equal once more.

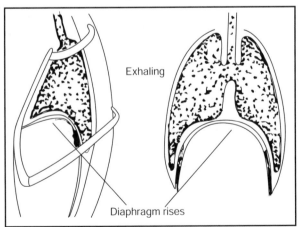

Figure 2:11. The diaphragm relaxes and rises during an exhalation, which causes air to leave the lungs.

Usually the same amount of air is breathed in and out, but it takes a little longer to exhale because breathing muscles are passive during this process. When breathing is no longer restful and muscles are used to actively exhale, such as when blowing out a candle, extra air is removed, which means that it will be necessary to take a deeper breath next time to equalise the pressure.

Gas Exchange in the Lungs

The alveoli are surrounded by tiny blood vessels called capillaries. The walls of both the alveoli and the capillaries are only one cell thick and because of this gases can pass through their walls, moving from the blood into the lungs and vice versa. The tension of oxygen in the alveoli (104 mm Hg) is greater than in the capillary blood (40 mm Hg) and so oxygen diffuses through the alveolar walls into the bloodstream to equalise pressure. The tension of carbon dioxide is greater in the capillaries (46 mm Hg) than in the alveoli (40 mm Hg), so it moves the other way (Tortora 1984).

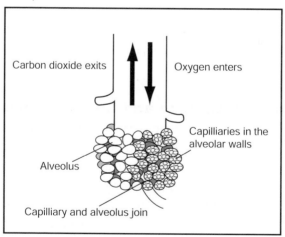

Figure 2:12. Gas exchange in the lungs.

Transporting Oxygen and Carbon Dioxide

Approximately 97% of the oxygen entering the bloodstream is carried through the body by haemoglobin molecules, which is found inside red blood cells. Each haemoglobin molecule is capable of carrying four oxygen molecules, and 100 mil of blood will normally carry 20 mil of oxygen.

Most of the carbon dioxide in the blood is transported back towards the lungs as bicarbonate ions, with only 20% carried by haemoglobin. However as it travels, carbon dioxide will switch back and forth between acidic and alkaline roles to balance the pH of the blood.

Gas Exchange in the Tissues

Like the alveoli, tissue cells have very thin walls and are surrounded by capillaries. Because of this the exchange of gases takes place once more here, only this time the exchange is in reverse with approximately one quarter of the oxygen carried by haemoglobin leaving the bloodstream and a considerable amount of carbon dioxide entering it. It requires only a single heartbeat to equalise the partial pressure of each gas in both the lungs and the tissues.

Reliance on Oxygen and Carbon Dioxide

It is easy to obtain adequate oxygen, and in fact most of the oxygen inhaled is simply breathed out again, which explains the ability to breathe for others who need resuscitating. Since it is possible to revive seriously ill people with less oxygen than is normally inhaled, it becomes obvious that high oxygen pressure is less important than is sometimes thought. In fact, it now appears that the higher percentage of carbon dioxide in the expired air may be beneficial to seriously ill people with acute respiratory distress syndrome (ARDS), acute inflammation and lack of oxygen to tissues, as recovery rate in hospitals has been shown to be faster when carbon dioxide pressure increases in the bloodstream (Hickling 1994, Laffey 1999).

In the tissue cells oxygen combines with a form of glucose called pyruvic acid to produce carbon dioxide, water and heat or energy.

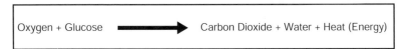

Figure 2:13. The production of carbon dioxide

This means that just by being alive, we continuously produce carbon dioxide, mostly in the working muscles. Because there is such a tiny amount of carbon dioxide in the atmosphere (0.04% of the total gas is carbon dioxide) and because gases move from high pressure to low pressure until the pressures are equal, it is easy to lose the carbon dioxide that is being produced. The atmosphere is so huge that it is impossible to make it equal the amount that is being breathed out, which is approximately 4.5% of the total exhaled air.

Scientists say that millions of years ago, before blue-green algae grew in the sea and forests covered the land, air on Earth was quite different to that of today (Lumb 2000). In fact it was similar to that of the atmosphere in the alveoli, meaning that a primeval - type atmosphere is retained inside the lungs. The developing baby in the womb grows in an environment that has an even higher tension of carbon dioxide (48 mm Hg) and less oxygen (30 mm Hg) than a baby who has been born (Lumb 2000), reinforcing the theory that carbon dioxide is more necessary for life than is generally thought possible.

Atmospheric air	
Oxygen	160mm Hg
Carbon Dioxide	0.3mm Hg
Alveolar section of the lungs	
Oxygen	105mm Hg
Carbon Dioxide	40mm Hg
Arterial or oxygenated blood	
Oxygen	105mm Hg
Carbon Dioxide	40mm Hg
Tissue cells	
Oxygen	40mm Hg
Carbon Dioxide	45mm Hg
Deoxygenated blood	
Oxygen	40mm Hg
Carbon Dioxide	45mm Hg
Exhaled air	
Oxygen	120mm Hg
Carbon Dioxide	27mm Hg

Table 2:1. Partial pressures of oxygen and carbon dioxide

Breathing Stimulation

There are four primary reasons why people breathe in a particular way:

1. To remove excess carbon dioxide from the bloodstream.
2. To ensure an adequate supply of oxygen to tissues
3. To regulate the pH of extracellular fluid (blood and other fluids found outside of tissue cells)
4. To maintain a steady internal or core temperature (Lum 1978).

Carbon Dioxide
Several chemical and physical reflexes regulate breathing, with

the most important of these for healthy people being the maintenance of carbon dioxide in the arteries at a constant pressure of 40 mm Hg (Tortora 1984). When a person is resting, the respiratory centre in the brain keeps this tension steady by maintaining breathing between four and six litres of air each minute. When the carbon dioxide pressure falls below 40 mm Hg then there is no stimulation of breathing and a moderate rhythmic pace is maintained until the pressure rises to 40 mm Hg again (Tortora 1984). But even a tiny increase in carbon dioxide tension stimulates breathing. For example if the tension rises by one mm Hg, an extra three litres of air is breathed each minute to rid the body of this excess (Kapit 2001).

During exercise, muscle cells require plenty of oxygen and consequently carbon dioxide is produced in large quantities. Now breathing speeds up or deepens dramatically to maintain the regular pressure, to the extent that healthy subjects have been measured at breathing over one hundred litres of air each minute (Grippi 1995). Similarly, a sudden drop in carbon dioxide pressure reduces the stimulation of breathing. By making these adjustments, the tension of carbon dioxide seldom varies by more than 3 mm Hg (Kapit 2001). However if breathing creates a change greater than this, the person is said to have dysfunctional breathing.

Oxygen
Low pressure of oxygen in the bloodstream stimulates breathing, but compared to carbon dioxide this is relatively rare. Approximately one hundred times less oxygen (1.55 litres) is stored in the body than carbon dioxide (120 litres), yet oxygen has to drop by over one third, from the standard 104 mm Hg to approximately 60 mm Hg, before breathing is stimulated to restore normal pressure (Lumb 2000). This indicates that survival is possible with considerably less oxygen than is ordinarily provided by breathing.

Arterial Blood pH

The maintenance of normal arterial blood pH is a third major stimulus for the breathing pattern as it is a constant survival instinct to maintain a pH of between 7.35 and 7.45. Carbon dioxide is the most important factor in keeping the pH regulated and is carried in many forms, such as carbon dioxide gas, carbonic acid and bicarbonates. Carbon dioxide itself is a weak acid and it easily combines with water to form carbonic acid. If blood becomes too acidic, carbonic acid breaks down to produce more bicarbonate ions to boost alkalinity, so by switching back and forth, the target pH of 7.4 is maintained.

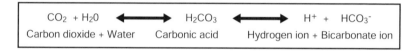

$$CO_2 + H_2O \longleftrightarrow H_2CO_3 \longleftrightarrow H^+ + HCO_3^-$$

Carbon dioxide + Water   Carbonic acid   Hydrogen ion + Bicarbonate ion

Figure 2:14. Balancing blood pH.

Because it is easy to retain or expel carbon dioxide, which is the basis of this cycle, by automatically altering the breathing, this is the primary way to keep blood within the healthy pH range. When blood becomes more acidic than usual, breathing escalates to rid the body of excess carbon dioxide; when blood becomes too alkaline, breathing is slowed to conserve it (Guyton 1982). If the problem is not corrected by breathing, then other adjustments are made, for example, the kidneys also play an important role in balancing pH by the adjustment of bicarbonates, or the excretion of lactic and keto acids. Breathing can make rapid changes to the pH, but compensation by the kidneys may take hours or even days (Guyton 1982).

Temperature

As body temperature increases, so does the breathing pattern, up to a certain point. For example, having a fever stimulates the breathing because like dogs we are able to cool ourselves by breathing faster.

The Bohr Effect

It is common knowledge that eating too much food does not mean good nutrition and this principle applies to breathing. Breathing too much air does not mean good breathing, nor does it even mean that extra oxygen is delivered to the tissues, because the amount of oxygen carried by the blood largely depends on haemoglobin content and the availability of oxygen rather than the depth of breathing. Providing the person is not anaemic and has healthy red blood cells there is no problem with haemoglobin, and unless the lungs are damaged, oxygen is readily available to the blood. Breathing calmly almost completely (98%) fills each haemoglobin cell with oxygen, so in theory it would only be possible to make a 2% improvement. However, since haemoglobin is constantly releasing oxygen, in reality it cannot be 100% saturated. Therefore breathing deeper is going to make virtually no improvement to the collection of oxygen by the haemoglobin.

Even when oxygen pressure dips from the average 104 mm Hg in the lungs to 60 mm Hg, haemoglobin is still 90% saturated with oxygen (Guyton 1982),so getting oxygen into the bloodstream is not usually the problem. Getting haemoglobin to release it is more of á challenge, because once haemoglobin and oxygen are joined, they form a tight bond and conditions need to be ideal in order for them to separate. This can be compared to four postage stamps joined together. It is always hard to tear off the first stamp, but once it has been removed, the other stamps come apart easily.

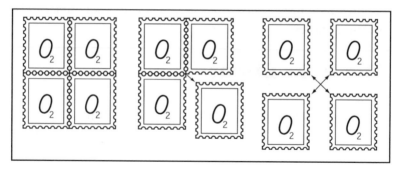

Figure 2:15. Haemoglobin and oxygen cling together like postage stamps.

In the early 20th century, Danish scientist Christian Bohr discovered that carbon dioxide pressure affects the ability of haemoglobin to carry oxygen (Lumb 2000). This is called the 'Bohr effect'. Low pressure of carbon dioxide means that oxygen is retained by haemoglobin and high pressure means that more oxygen is released to tissue cells. Temperature and low oxygen pressure in tissue cells also drive oxygen off haemoglobin. The body is like a well-balanced machine - when it is working hard and the tissue cells need extra oxygen, it is simultaneously making an abundance of carbon dioxide and heat, thus ensuring a steady flow of oxygen to the tissues.

A problem can occur however, when breathing is increased to the level where too much carbon dioxide is exhaled. This compels blood to become more alkaline than normal (Respiratory Alkalosis) and haemoglobin becomes 'stickier', retaining oxygen instead of releasing it. This creates a vicious circle, because less oxygen reaching tissues means that less carbon dioxide is being produced.

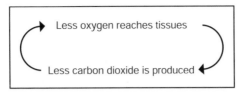

Figure 2:16. The production of carbon dioxide and the release of oxygen are dependent on each other.

The graph below of the Bohr effect shows the connection between oxygen release and carbon dioxide pressure.

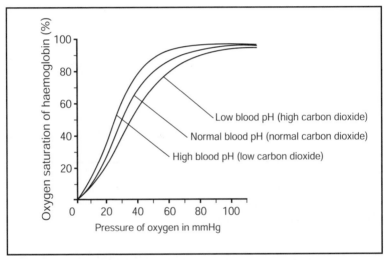

Figure 2:17. The Bohr effect and its consequence on oxygen tension. When blood is less alkaline, more oxygen is released from haemoglobin and received by the tissues.

The Reality of the Bohr Effect

On a basic and practical level the Bohr effect means that in spite of oxygen content in the blood being normal, when more air is breathed than is required tissue cells are starved of oxygen. Breathing quietly and steadily actually means better oxygenation because adequate supplies of both oxygen and carbon dioxide are maintained. This scientific fact is totally the opposite from the way the person feels when short of breath.

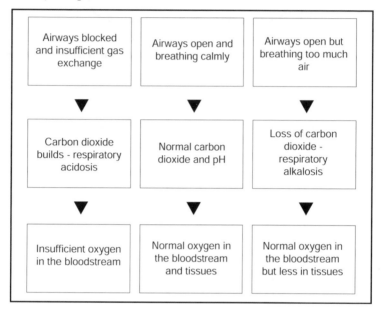

Figure 2:18. When the person breathes calmly sufficient oxygen both reaches the lungs and is released to tissues. Not breathing enough or breathing too much will cause a problem.

It is accepted that when smoking a cigarette less oxygen is available to tissues and this is one of the reasons that smokers generally have older looking skin than nonsmokers. Because of the Bohr effect, breathing more air than is required for metabolism is also going to mean that less oxygen is released to tissues and this might be done for several hours a day, if not continuously. So for a lengthy time each day, just like a cigarette smoker, slightly less oxygen will be reaching tissues. When tissues do not receive sufficient oxygen, lactic acid is produced by and accumulates in the tissue (Fried 1993), which makes them ache and tire quickly. It also makes the whole body feel tired and lacking in energy. One more factor to consider is that everyone has an organ or tissues that are genetically weaker than they should be and these are likely to show the first sign of wear and tear, or to suffer the most from a lack of oxygen. This may help to explain why there is such a wide range of symptoms associated with hyperventilation.

References

Anderson Price S, McCarty Wilson L. Pathophysiology. Clinical concepts of Disease Processes. Fourth Edition. Mosby. St. Louis. 1992. p260

Buteyko KP. Private interview circa 1980.

Fried R. The Psychology and Physiology of Breathing. Plenum Press. New York 1993. p104

Grippi M. Pulmonary Pathophysiology. J.B. Lippincott Company. Philadelphia. 1995. p287

Guyton. AC. Human Physiology and Mechanisms of Disease. W.B. Saunders Co. Philadelphia. 1982. pp279-280, 285, 300, 306, 320-323

Henderson. Y. Cyclopedia of Medicine. 1940

Hickling KG, Walsh J, Henderson S, Jackson R. Low mortality rate in adult respiratory distress syndrome using low-volume, pressure-limited ventilation with permissive hypercapnia: a prospective study. Critical Care Medicine. 1994. 22. pp1568-1578

Kapit W, Macey RI, Meisami E. The Physiology Colouring Book. Addison Wesley Longman Inc. San Francisco. 2001. p56

Laffey JG, Kavanagh BP. Carbon dioxide and the critically ill – too little of a good thing? Lancet. 1999. 354(9186). pp1283-1286

Lum LC. Respiratory Alkalosis and Hypocarbia. The roles of carbon dioxide in the body economy. Chest, Heart & Stroke. Winter 1978/79. 3(4). pp31-34

Lumb AB. Nunn's Applied Respiratory Physiology. Reed. London. 2000. pp 3-12, 237, 267, 321, 362

Naifeh K. Behavioural and Psychological Approaches to Breathing Disorders. Ed. B.H. Timmons & R Ley. Plenum. New York. 1994. p17

Piper AJ, Parker S, Torzillo PJ et al. Nocturnal nasal IPPV stabilizes patients with CF and hypercapnic respiratory failure. Chest 1992. 102. pp846-850

Tortora GJ, Anagnostakos NP. Principles of Anatomy and Physiology, Harper & Row, New York. 1984. pp562 563, 564, 570, 587, 693

Chapter 3

Hyperventilation

Buteyko Practitioners use the Bohr effect to challenge and demonstrate how traditional ideas on breathing, such as oxygen being the 'good' gas and carbon dioxide the 'bad', are incorrect. If oxygen is 'good' for human life, then the ideal atmosphere would be 100% oxygen, yet according to textbooks (Guyton, 1982 for example), breathing pure oxygen has been shown to cause blindness in babies (retrolental fibroplasia) and it is also detrimental to the nervous system, sometimes causing epileptic seizures and coma, or at the very least large concentrations of free radicals, which can damage the metabolic system of tissue cells.

In spite of the evidence to the contrary, western society has an established misconception that deep breathing is beneficial. For example, several forms of relaxation techniques incorporate deep breathing into their regimes in the belief that it improves both oxygenation and health, while simultaneously reducing stress levels. These ideas are further compounded by the notion that mucus is something that must be removed, instead of a natural secretion that protects and lubricates the airways. The following are examples of misconceptions about breathing:

- 'Deep breathing is relaxing and gives you more oxygen.'
- 'You breathe in oxygen and breathe out carbon dioxide.'
- 'Have a good cough and get rid of that mucus.'
- 'Chest out, tummy in!'
- 'Hyperventilation means taking big, deep breaths.'

These thoughts are based on perception rather than fact. For example, mouth-to-mouth resuscitation would be impossible if only carbon dioxide is breathed out, and deep breathing is not at all relaxing during a panic attack.

In the past from time to time it has been stylish for women to have 'wasp waists' or 'hour glass' figures. Since most women are not naturally built this way, the effect was achieved by wearing corsets that pulled in the abdomen so tightly that the women were forced to breathe with their upper chest muscles instead of their diaphragm. Upper chest muscles are normally only used during vigorous exercise and since most of the time these women seldom did serious physical work, they were continuously breathing more than they needed to. As soon as their breathing rate increased a little more, perhaps at the thought of something shocking or exciting, less oxygen reached the brain and they 'had a fit of the vapours', or fainted. If history can be believed, during these times women (at least those of the privileged classes) were considered delicate creatures, many being semi-invalids who spent a great deal of time resting, which is no wonder when fashion forced them to breathe incorrectly for most of their adult life.

Two Types of Hyperventilation

There are two types of hyperventilation – acute and chronic. Acute hyperventilation has profound symptoms that most people can relate to; the light-headed feeling after blowing up several balloons, or 'butterflies' in the stomach and feeling weak at the knees before going on stage are classic examples.

Acute Hyperventilation

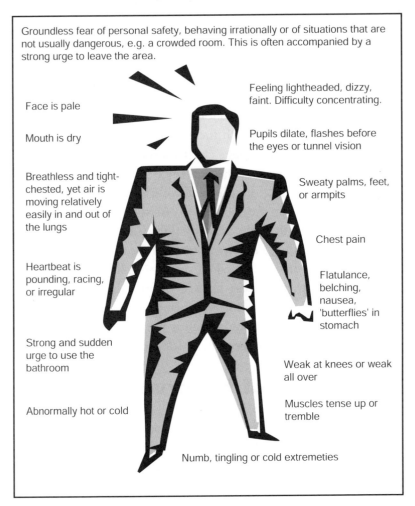

Groundless fear of personal safety, behaving irrationally or of situations that are not usually dangerous, e.g. a crowded room. This is often accompanied by a strong urge to leave the area.

Face is pale

Mouth is dry

Breathless and tight-chested, yet air is moving relatively easily in and out of the lungs

Heartbeat is pounding, racing, or irregular

Strong and sudden urge to use the bathroom

Abnormally hot or cold

Feeling lightheaded, dizzy, faint. Difficulty concentrating.

Pupils dilate, flashes before the eyes or tunnel vision

Sweaty palms, feet, or armpits

Chest pain

Flatulance, belching, nausea, 'butterflies' in stomach

Weak at knees or weak all over

Muscles tense up or tremble

Numb, tingling or cold extremeties

Figure 3:1. Acute Hyperventilation causes many diverse symptoms. The person however, may not always link the symptoms to their breathing.

The following list of symptoms of **acute hyperventilation** have been adapted from a variety of sources, namely the Agoraphobic Program Treatment Manual of St. Vincent's Hospital, Sydney Australia (1982), Behavioral and Psychological Approaches to Breathing Disorders (1994) and The Psychology and Physiology of Breathing (1993):

Shortness of breath; chest tightness; chest pain (not heart-related); light-headedness or dizziness; feeling faint; lack of concentration; numbness, tingling or cold extremities; heartbeat that is irregular, pounding or racing; fear that you will do something crazy, lose control or die; anxiety; tension; apprehension, urge to escape; irritability; dry mouth; digestive tract dysfunction (e.g. flatulence, belching, nausea, diarrhoea); visual disturbances (e.g. dilated pupils, flashes before the eyes, tunnel vision); muscle spasm or trembling; feeling suddenly hot or cold; sweaty palms or feet; and general weakness. In severe cases, loss of consciousness may occur.

Chronic Hyperventilation

The second type of hyperventilation is **chronic or habitual** and is more often than not caused by the prolonged, low grade stress of overeating, lack of exercise, overuse of stimulants (e.g. coffee, soft drinks, cigarettes) and exposure to pollutants, all of which have become an almost daily occurrence in the developed world.

When the shoulders are heaving, chest is rising rapidly or the breathing is noisy, it is easy to think 'Hyperventilation!" Chronic hyperventilation however, does not usually mean any of these things. Instead breathing may be a little faster than usual, using the upper chest muscles instead of the diaphragm or perhaps breathing at a normal rate through the nose most of the time with a deep breath, yawn or sigh every few minutes.

Most of the symptoms are less sharp than those of acute hyperventilation, but no less real and certainly evident. All parts of the body can be affected, which can create dismay, and confusion as to what is wrong.

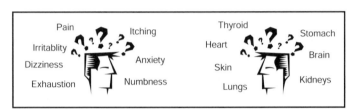

The following list has been compiled from researchers Innocenti (1997), Lum (1977), Magarian (1982) and Timmons (1994):

Shortness of breath; chest tightness; extra-sensitive airways; excessive production of mucus resulting in frequent sneezing, coughing, nose-blowing, repeated throat clearing, long term blocked or running sinus; frequent yawning and sighing; light-headedness, dizziness, unsteadiness, feeling 'spaced out'; poor concentration; numbness, tingling and coldness especially in the hands, feet and face; heartbeat that is irregular, pounding or racing; degrees of anxiety, tension, phobias, depression, irritability and apprehension; dry mouth; digestive disorders - abdominal bloating, belching, flatulence, diarrhoea, constipation; tiredness, general weakness, chronic exhaustion; poor sleep patterns; chest pain (not heart-related); pale or itchy skin; sweaty palms; sore muscles, cramps; tremor; headaches.

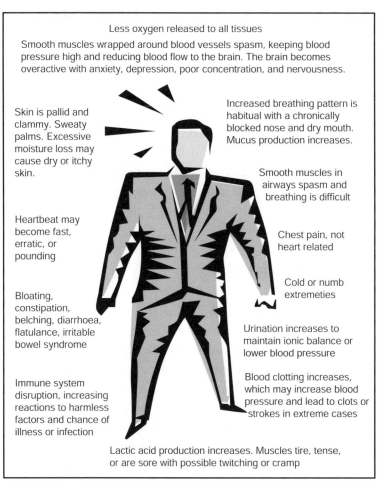

Less oxygen released to all tissues

Smooth muscles wrapped around blood vessels spasm, keeping blood pressure high and reducing blood flow to the brain. The brain becomes overactive with anxiety, depression, poor concentration, and nervousness.

Skin is pallid and clammy. Sweaty palms. Excessive moisture loss may cause dry or itchy skin.

Increased breathing pattern is habitual with a chronically blocked nose and dry mouth. Mucus production increases.

Smooth muscles in airways spasm and breathing is difficult

Heartbeat may become fast, erratic, or pounding

Chest pain, not heart related

Bloating, constipation, belching, diarrhoea, flatulance, irritable bowel syndrome

Cold or numb extremeties

Urination increases to maintain ionic balance or lower blood pressure

Immune system disruption, increasing reactions to harmless factors and chance of illness or infection

Blood clotting increases, which may increase blood pressure and lead to clots or strokes in extreme cases

Lactic acid production increases. Muscles tire, tense, or are sore with possible twitching or cramp

Figure 3:2. Chronic hyperventilation is subtle, but not the symptoms.

In addition to these symptoms, others can occur of which the person is totally unaware, such as a depressed immune response or blood vessels withdrawing from the skin and blood thickening to prevent potential bleeding. While this is useful for a short sprint away from danger, it is not so useful in a world of continual stresses, as the skin may now continually be less nourished or the blood more prone to clotting.

The Carbon Dioxide Syndrome

The Carbon Dioxide Syndrome is a condition where the person has chronic hyperventilation, and very often acute as well. This means that the symptoms are usually moderate, with the more alarming kind happening from time to time. The increased level of breathing is not usually obvious at first glance unless you are specifically looking for it, which is typical of any form of hyperventilation. Even though breathing is the most crucial survival requirement and affects every organ and cell in the human body, it is largely taken for granted and ignored until it becomes seriously altered.

Good Breathing

Good breathing means breathing sufficient air to meet the demands of metabolism and no more. Along with food, oxygen provides energy to meet the demands of metabolism so that the body functions properly. Imagine that eating one bar of chocolate and breathing fourteen times a minute provides sufficient energy to walk for one hour. If someone eats two bars of chocolate but still only walks for one hour, then he or she has eaten more calories than are required to complete the walk. This is eating more than is required for metabolic demands and will cause a weight gain if it is continued. Breathing thirty times a minute while taking the same walk is breathing more than is required for normal metabolism, and like eating the two bars of chocolate, it is only a minor change but one that will eventually cause a problem if it is maintained.

When breathing correctly, the breathing is:

- Quiet and soft during sleep and rest.
- Comfortable through the nose almost all the time.
- Still easy to do while exercising.

And *not*

- Feeling restricted.
- Blowing the nose repeatedly.
- Coughing excessively.

How many people breathe like this? Do you?

Take the Hyperventilation Test

The symptoms of hyperventilation often appear totally unrelated to breathing. For example sweaty palms or feeling 'spaced out' do not appear to have any direct link with moving air in and out of the body, yet they are commonly associated with dysfunctional breathing.

To check how likely it is that you hyperventilate, take the following test and rate yourself on a scale of 0 - 4 for the following symptoms, where:

0 is never
1 is rare
2 is sometimes
3 is often
4 is very often.

0 1 2 3 4	Airways are extra-sensitive
0 1 2 3 4	Allergies, rhinitis, hay fever
0 1 2 3 4	Bloated abdomen, flatulence or belching
0 1 2 3 4	Breathing erratically. E.g. taking a deep breath every few minutes; breathing without pause; rapid breathing spaced with long pauses
0 1 2 3 4	Breathing that is frequently fast or deep
0 1 2 3 4	Breathing through mouth
0 1 2 3 4	Chest constriction or tightness
0 1 2 3 4	Chest pains that are not heart-related
0 1 2 3 4	Cold hands or feet
0 1 2 3 4	Colds, flu or chest infections
0 1 2 3 4	Constipation with intermittent diarrhoea
0 1 2 3 4	Coughing
0 1 2 3 4	Dental or gum problems
0 1 2 3 4	Depression
0 1 2 3 4	Difficulty in taking a deep breath
0 1 2 3 4	Dry mouth
0 1 2 3 4	Headaches
0 1 2 3 4	Heartbeat that pounds or is rapid or erratic
0 1 2 3 4	High blood pressure
0 1 2 3 4	Irritability or short temper
0 1 2 3 4	Itchy or dry skin
0 1 2 3 4	Licking dry lips
0 1 2 3 4	Light-headed or dizzy
0 1 2 3 4	Loss of libido
0 1 2 3 4	Mucus production that is excessive
0 1 2 3 4	Muscle tightness or cramps
0 1 2 3 4	Nose that blocks regularly
0 1 2 3 4	Pains in bones
0 1 2 3 4	Physical exhaustion, lack of stamina, chronic tiredness
0 1 2 3 4	Poor concentration, mental fatigue, confusion

0 1 2 3 4   Sense of smell is reduced
0 1 2 3 4   Short of breath
0 1 2 3 4   Sighing when you are not harassed
0 1 2 3 4   Sinuses that continually block or drain
0 1 2 3 4   Sleeping badly e.g. insomnia, vivid dreams,
             nightmares, shuddering in sleep, snoring,
             waking frequently, grinding teeth or still feeling
             tired after a long sleep
0 1 2 3 4   Stiffness in fingers or arms
0 1 2 3 4   Sweaty palms/feet/armpits or generally feeling
             hot all over
0 1 2 3 4   Tension, apprehension, anxiety, panic or fear
             without reason e.g. fear of stuffy rooms
0 1 2 3 4   Throat clearing repeatedly
0 1 2 3 4   Tightness around the mouth
0 1 2 3 4   Tingling or numb extremities
             (e.g. fingers or lips)
0 1 2 3 4   Trembling and tic
0 1 2 3 4   Upper chest breathing
0 1 2 3 4   Visual disturbances e.g. flashes or shadows
             before the eyes, blurred or tunnel vision or
             impaired night vision
0 1 2 3 4   Yawning when you are not tired

Total _____

The maximum score for this test is 180 and it is doubtful that
you would have completed it if your breathing warranted such a
high score. However, a rating of '3' for ten of these symptoms
indicates a tendency towards having the Carbon Dioxide
Syndrome, and the more symptoms that you scored, the worse
your problem is likely to be.

Why Hyperventilation Produces Symptoms

Hyperventilation cannot provide a lot more oxygen than normal breathing, but it *always* removes too much carbon dioxide, firstly from the lungs and then the bloodstream (Anderson Price 1992, Tortora 1984). When carbon dioxide becomes low in the bloodstream a number of things happen, which include:

- Less oxygen is delivered to all parts of the body because of the Bohr effect (Anderson Price 1982).
- The blood becomes more alkaline than usual (Respiratory Alkalosis) and alkalosis not only affects oxygen delivery but it also interferes with the removal of calcium from red blood cells and muscles. The build-up of calcium enhances the ability of all muscles to spasm, as well as making red blood cells more rigid and the nervous system particularly excitable (Brewer 1974, Brody 1932, Levine 1984, Naifeh 1994, Yasue 1980).
- Smooth muscle spasms. Smooth or involuntary muscle is wrapped around all the hollow places in the body, such as blood vessels, airways, digestive tract, fallopian tubes, womb, bladder, bowel, and parts of all organs. Unlike skeletal muscle, smooth muscle is not under conscious control. Instead it is affected by other factors such as low pressure of carbon dioxide, which causes it to restrict the flow or movement of automatic processes. For example, blood flow to both the brain and the body's extremities is reduced, with the brain being particularly affected.
- Histamine production increases. Histamine is a chemical that the body uses to attack and restrict the movement of foreign particles that have either entered the body or come in contact with the skin. Its presence causes a variety of

reactions such as a rash, swelling, heat, an increase in mucus production and also spasm of smooth muscle (Kontos 1972).

To summarise: breathing affects every cell in the body by supplying oxygen and removing carbon dioxide. Acute hyperventilation is likely to cause extreme symptoms such as dizziness and fear. And while the symptoms of chronic hyperventilation are less obvious, it is not doing the body any good either. The body is both directly affected by oxygen deprivation for example, or is compensating in some way to deal with the disturbance chronic hyperventilation causes. Either way the body functions less effectively.

Why Breathing Becomes Abnormal

Hyperventilation is a natural response to stress, which literally means *any* stress. The type of stress that humans have evolved to best cope with is the relatively short-lived and physical kind, such as digging the garden. Hyperventilation that is caused by a stressful desk job is not easy to cope with because it is prolonged, requires little physical activity, and until very recent history, was not something that people normally had to do day after day.

Such little attention is paid to breathing that the normal rate can easily double before being noticed (Coope 1948) and even the symptoms of acute hyperventilation are often not attributed to the breathing pattern. In fact, they usually occur when the person is doing something that is stimulating but has little physical activity, such as driving a car, watching television or simply being in a crowded room, rather than while breathing vigorously when blowing up balloons (Lum 1994). It is not possible to *acutely* hyperventilate for a lengthy period because when insufficient oxygen reaches the brain due to this kind of breathing, the person faints. Immediately the brain releases calming opiates that slow the breathing, oxygen is restored and the person wakes up again (Fried 1993).

It is however, possible to *chronically* hyperventilate at a low grade because the body is adaptive. For example, at altitude there is less air, yet people can still live there because the body compensates for the lower oxygen level by increasing haemoglobin content, volume of blood, number of blood vessels, heart size and also by the amount of air breathed each minute (Guyton 1982). The extra breathing has the additional effect of lowering carbon dioxide pressure. Similarly, when any other kind of stress is constant and less carbon dioxide is found in the bloodstream, the body also adapts as it would if you lived at altitude (Jennet 1994). This adaptive ability allows the respiratory centre to maintain a breathing pattern that is slightly faster or deeper than it used to be *all* the time, so that it can maintain this new lowered pressure of carbon dioxide.

When the person first begins to hyperventilate and to disturb their pH and carbon dioxide pressure, the respiratory centre attempts to deal with it by not stimulating the breathing, instead it is quiet and unhurried. However, if this is not sufficient to maintain homoeostasis, then the nose might become stuffy or the airways constrict slightly, in a greater effort to conserve carbon dioxide.

If these measures are also inadequate, two things might happen:
>   1. More drastic narrowing of the airways occurs to avoid
>   an even greater loss of carbon dioxide.

2. The body begins to adapt to the changed pressure by making adjustments in other areas, creating metabolic acidosis for example.

This is because basically there is no real mechanism to prevent the pressure of carbon dioxide from dropping, unlike the opposite (Gardner 1994). When carbon dioxide rises, breathing is directly stimulated until the pressure drops back to normal; but when the pressure is low, breathing becomes more passive but it still continues.

The following scenario about "Bill" is an example of how this could happen: For Bill, life is great. He enjoys excellent health and has a wonderful job. His body continuously produces carbon dioxide and he breathes five litres of air each minute while resting to maintain a healthy pressure of 40 mm Hg in the arterial blood.

Then one year Bill catches the flu and is sick for three weeks. During this time his temperature is high, pulse is rapid and his nose is blocked, all of which causes him to breathe ten litres of air each minute. Most of the time he sleeps or watches television and because his breathing is constantly more than is needed for these activities, carbon dioxide tension drops. Because his respiratory centre is not able to maintain the normal pressure of 40 mm Hg, it adjusts to 38 mm Hg.

Even when well again and taking part in everyday activities, Bill's brain maintains this new pressure by making him breathe eight litres of air each minute. There are no obvious signs of hyperventilation, but from time to time when life gets a little hectic, he gets some hay fever or eczema. When subjected to other long-term stress, Bill's respiratory centre adapts again to the slightly lowered tension of carbon dioxide and constantly increases the breathing pattern to maintain it. Now he gets sinus headaches, more hay fever and feels anxious from time to time for no particular reason.

Other kinds of stress that may not involve a lot of physical activity include excitement and anticipation, getting sick, going on holiday, expecting visitors, or playing a variation of a game that children have been playing for centuries. This game involves some 'hide and seek' with a lot of running and simulated fighting. It is exciting as the children try to evade capture or capture others and today's children also play this game, but more often than not it is played on a computer. This is just as exciting, but there is one vital component missing, it does not involve any actual running. The extra breathing associated with the game when it is completely unnecessary for the amount of physical activity being exerted – only pushing buttons or manipulating a joystick - is one way of permanently altering the breathing pattern if it is played often enough or for a lengthy time.

Once the brain has adapted to a lower pressure of carbon dioxide, it is easy to keep it low because chronic hyperventilation frequently goes undetected (Anderson Price 1992). This is for a number of reasons that may include:

- Breathing is automatic and scarcely noticed until it is extreme, for example taking 12 breaths of air per minute of 0.5 litre of air equals 6 litres and 20 breaths of 0.75 litre equals 15 litres, more than doubling the amount with virtually no effort or obvious difference.
- Hyperventilation is frequently intermittent with periods of normal breathing in between. For example, people seldom snore *all* night, but do so on and off.

- *One* single deep breath will reduce carbon dioxide by approximately 6% or between 7 and 16 mm Hg. (Anderson Price 1992; Engel et al 1947; Fried 1981 and Rowbottom 1992).

The 'Mimic' and 'Fat Folder' Syndrome

Chronic hyperventilation is sometimes called 'Hyperventilation Syndrome' or 'Chronic Hyperventilation Syndrome'. In this book it is mostly referred to as the 'Carbon Dioxide Syndrome' and others call it 'The Mimic' or the 'Fat Folder Syndrome' because nearly all the symptoms of hyperventilation can be found in other illnesses or diseases. For example, a common symptom of hyperventilation – both acute and chronic, is to feel short of breath. Any number of other states may also make you feel this way; asthma, emphysema, heart conditions, lung cancer, pneumonia and simply being unfit are just a few of them.

Lum (1975) reports that sometimes the sole problem is hyperventilation but the symptoms have been given another name, which is hyperventilation being 'The Mimic'. In an extreme case he cites a man who underwent open-heart surgery for his 'black outs'. The surgery was of no benefit and the man continued to have black outs until he addressed his hyperventilation with a respiratory physiotherapist. Since the average person cannot tell whether there is something seriously wrong or not, they visit their doctor who organises 'some tests'. In the case of hyperventilation-related chest pain for example, the tests come back negative because the symptoms have no organic basis, however the person still has the pain. Now the worry is (a) 'It's all in the mind', and there is concern about being a hypochondriac, or (b) there is something seriously wrong which has not yet been diagnosed.

has not yet been diagnosed.

Both of these situations are likely to create more stress and consequently more hyperventilation, which either makes the current symptoms worse or causes new ones to appear. The person is sent for still more tests, all of which reveal nothing of significance, but because there are so many test results the person's medical file grows larger, hence the 'Fat Folder Syndrome' (Fensterheim 1994).

'I wasn't hyperventilating, I wasn't an asthmatic. I kept saying to myself. Boy did I get a surprise! Now I know that I've been running on three cylinders all that time and it sure feels great to be running on four again. What a difference. If your car doesn't run well you get it fixed. Book yourself into a Buteyko course, you won't regret it.' Antje

References

Anderson Price S, McCarty Wilson L. Pathophysiology. Clinical concepts of Disease Processes. Fourth Edition. Mosby St. Louis. 1992. pp271, 539

Brewer GJ. Red cell metabolism and function. In the Red Cell. Ed. G M Surgeon. New York Academic Press. 1974

Brody BS and Dusser de Barenne JGD. Effect of hyperventilation of the excitability of the motor cortex in cats. Arch Neurol Psychiat 1932. 28. pp571-585

Coope Robert. Diseases of the Chest. E & S Livingstone. 1948. p48

Engel GL., Ferris EB, Logan M. Hyperventilation: Analysis of clinical symptomatology. Annals of Internal Medicine. 1947. pp683–704

Fensterheim H. Behavioural and Psychological Approaches to Breathing Disorders. Ed. B.H. Timmons & R Ley. Plenum. New York. 1994. p143

Fried R. The Hyperventilation Syndrome Research and Clinical Treatment. The John Hopkins University Press. 1987. p41

Fried R. The Psychology and Physiology of Breathing. Plenum Press. New York 1993. pp214-215

Gardner WN. Behavioural and Psychological Approaches to Breathing Disorders. Ed. B.H. Timmons & R Ley. Plenum. New York. 1994. p101

Guyton. AC. Human Physiology and Mechanisms of Disease. W.B. Saunders Co. Philadelphia. 1982. pp333, 336

Innocenti. DM. Cash's Text Book for Physiotherapists. Chest, Heart and Cardiovascular Conditions. Faber and Faber 1997. p449

Jennet S. Behavioural and Psychological Approaches to Breathing Disorders. Ed. B.H. Timmons & R Ley. Plenum. New York. 1994. p77

Kontos HA, Richardson DW, Raper AJ, Zubair-Ul-Hassan, Patterson JL. Mechanisms of action of hypocapnic alkalosis on limb blood vessels in man and dog. Am J Physiology. Dec 1972. 223. pp1296-1307

Levine BS, Coburn JW. Magnesium, the mimic/antagonist of calcium. N Engl J Medicine. 1984. 310. pp1253-1255

Lum LC. Behavioural and Psychological Approaches to Breathing Disorders. Ed. B.H. Timmons & R Ley. Plenum. New York. 1994. p116

Lum, LC. Breathing Exercises in the Treatment of Hyperventilation and Chronic Anxiety States. Chest, Heart & Stroke Journal. Spring 1977. 2. p1

Lum LC. Hyperventilation: The tip and the iceberg. J Psychosom Res. 1975. 19. pp375-383

Magarian GJ. Hyperventilation Syndromes: Infrequently Recognized Common Expressions of Anxiety and Stress. Medicine. The Williams and Wilkins Co. 1982. 61(4). pp219-236

Naifeh K. Behavioural and Psychological Approaches to Breathing Disorders. Ed. B.H. Timmons & R Ley. Plenum. New York. 1994. p29

Rowbottom I. The physiotherapy management of chronic hyperventilation. ACPRC. 1992. 21. pp9-12

Timmons BH. Behavioural and Psychological Approaches to Breathing Disorders. Ed. B.H. Timmons & R Ley. Plenum. New York. 1994. p4

The Agoraphobic Program Treatment Manual. St. Vincent's Hospital, Sydney. 1993. p3

Tortora GJ, Anagnostakos NP. Principles of Anatomy and Physiology, Harper & Row, New York. 1984. p693

Yasue H. Pathophysiology and treatment of coronary arterial spasm. Chest. 1980. 78. pp216 – 233

Chapter 4

Nose v Mouth

Until at least six months old, a baby virtually always breathes through its nose, which is important for survival because sucking for several minutes is the normal way of feeding. Even when crawling and learning to walk, a healthy baby still breathes through its nose and uses the diaphragm rather than the upper chest. In fact, babies do not generally breathe through their mouths unless they are sick or crying.

It is less socially acceptable for an adult to walk around with their mouth hanging open than it is for a child, but once mouth breathing becomes habitual in childhood it is not easy to break the habit. There are three major reasons for this:

- The respiratory centre in the brain has adapted to an abnormally low pressure of carbon dioxide and nose breathing quickly raises the pressure, which stimulates the breathing.
- If medications are used to open up the nasal passages for any length of time, there is frequently a rebound effect that causes the nose to block even more, causing an increased sense of claustrophobia or 'lacking in air'.
- There is not always a comfortable amount of room for the tongue within the mouth cavity.

People are born with a particular shaped head, but the way a child breathes directly shapes the skull as it grows because the tongue rests on the roof of the mouth when a person breathes through his nose, acting like a natural retainer. If this is the habit as a child, the palate, nasal passages, and the entire face widen into the typical oval shape. When the child breathes through their mouth, the tongue rests on the floor of the mouth instead of the roof and the natural broadening of the face is less likely to occur. If this kind of breathing is habitual, the face becomes more narrow or elongated compared to that of nose-breathing siblings (Champagne 1991, Rubin 1980). By the time the tongue has grown to full size, the mouth cavity may be so small that there is little room for the tongue to fit into the closed mouth. This can make breathing through the mouth almost a necessity.

Nose-Breathing

Because the nose is smaller than the mouth, less air is inhaled when it is breathed through, and this smaller volume of air is travelling at the ideal speed to be warmed, moistened and cleaned before it reaches the lungs (Guyton 1982). Within the nasal passages tiny hairs and mucus help to trap irritants such as dust and pollen and the air also becomes germfree as it flows past the adenoid and tonsil filters. Mucus also contains a chemical called lysozyme that kills bacteria, adding to the protection that nose breathing provides. The nose is so effective at filtration that even though approximately 500 litres of air are breathed each hour, most of the microbes in the air never even reach the trachea (Coope 1948).

The nose creates a definite pressure difference between the lungs and the atmosphere, improving airflow and an extra 10 - 20% oxygen is diffused into the bloodstream (Cottle 1972).

The improvement in efficiency of the lungs means the heart also works more effectively, ensuring more oxygen reaches tissues.

Breathing Through the Mouth

The mouth does not warm or moisten inhaled air and so large gulps of cold and dry air reach the lungs. The air is also not cleaned properly because there are no hairs, mucus blanket, or adenoids to collect germs.

People with breathing problems have sometimes been taught to breathe through their mouth – doing 'pursed lip' breathing, which is where the exhalation is a soft whistle. Any kind of mouth breathing lowers airflow resistance causing the lungs to function less efficiently. Consequently less oxygen reaches the bloodstream, making the heart work a little harder. Apart from making the airways stay open a little longer while exhaling, pursed lip breathing is not useful because it causes a greater loss of water vapour and carbon dioxide, while disrupting cardiac output and blood flow in the chest. This means that it takes more energy to breathe like this, so you actually need more oxygen to do it (Hough 1997).

Chronic mouth-breathing can also contribute to:

- Headache
- Head bent forward, which can lead to neck or back muscle pain, stiffness, fatigue or cervical joint damage
- Dry mouth and throat
- Chronic tonsil swelling
- Enlarged adenoids and polyps
- Chronic cough and/or throat clearing
- Noisy breathing

- Noisy eating
- Impaired sense of smell
- Snoring
- Sleep apnoea
- Extra mucus production
- Bloating, flatulence, belching

(Davies 1989, Hough 1997, Magarian 1982).

Breathing through the mouth also causes or contributes to the following dental problems:

- Dental decay
- Gum disease
- Malocclusion (teeth not fitting together properly when the mouth is shut)
- Anterior open bite (prominent top teeth)
- Reduced dental arch space (narrow roof of the mouth.)
- Greater potential for relapse of orthodontic correction
- TMJ (where the jaw bone hinges onto cheek bone) dysfunction
- Bad breath

(Coventry 2000, Guyton 1982).

The narrow palate caused by habitual mouth breathing as a child generally leads to teeth that either overlap or move forward, making a large overbite. As it is not possible to chew, swallow or even talk properly, orthodontic work and tooth removal are required to correct the bite. Teeth will wear unevenly if treatment is not performed early, resulting in dental work being required later in life.

Nose-breathing is also important for the health of teeth and gums even when the teeth are well spaced, because it ensures a greater supply of saliva. Saliva keeps the mouth healthy by protecting it against bacterial infection and tooth erosion from acids (Guyton 1982). Bacteria are either inhaled through the mouth or enter with food and fingers for example. Acids arrive in the mouth via eating and drinking or as a result of gastric reflux. Breathing through the mouth dries out the protective saliva and can also easily cause dehydration, which is the most common source of salivary dysfunction (Dawes 1987).

Breathing through the mouth and using asthma medication increases the danger of tooth decay even further because reliever medication stifles saliva production (McDerra 1998, Shaw 2000, Ryberg 1987). Some asthma medications are acidic, which is another reason for possible damage to the teeth (O'Sullivan 1998). Steroid puffers decrease immune system efficiency and encourage the growth of oral thrush (Wilson 2002), clearly not promoting a healthy environment for teeth and gums.

Conclusion

Breathing through the nose with very little bodily movement is the natural, healthy way while resting. There is no good reason why a person needs to breathe any other way unless there is physical damage to the nasal passages. From an aesthetic point of view, breathing through your nose makes life nicer; you can smell the roses, taste the food and enjoy that glass of wine much more, so there seems little to recommend breathing through the mouth, apart from the fact that it is easier to do when quantity of air seems more important than quality.

Getting Your Nose Clear

Many people find it difficult to breathe through their nose because the nose is one of those things that the saying, 'If you don't use it, you lose it', applies to. It is often thought that if you breathe through your mouth it is because your nose blocked up first, but typically the nose blocks after you start breathing through your mouth and because it is uncomfortable breathing through a stuffy nose, after a while you stop trying. Once mouth-breathing has become an established habit, it takes a lot of effort to retrain yourself to breathe through your nose.

The first step to take is to get your nose clear enough to breathe through, so try the following exercise which will help to make your nose easier to breathe through:

- Sit on a straight-backed chair.
- After a normal breath out, close your mouth (if it was open), and softly pinch the end of your nose to seal the nostrils.
- Gently and slowly nod your head up and down six to eight times.
- Keep your mouth closed and take your hand off your nose, allowing the nostrils to open.
- Breathe *softly* and *gently* through your nose, while still keeping your mouth closed.
- Providing the nasal passages have opened slightly, continue to breathe gently through your nose.

If your nose is not totally clear, take another two or three breaths before repeating the exercise. It may be repeated several times in order to completely clear your nose.

If you cannot get your nose to clear by using this exercise, then sucking peppermints or taking nasal steroids for a short period may also give you temporary relief which will assist the clearing of your nose. If these measures do not help, then ask your doctor to check your nasal passages for the presence of polyps or other blockages so that you can get your nose working as effectively as possible.

'My doctor advised me to see an ear, nose and throat specialist in order to be operated on for correction of an alleged deviation in my nasal septum. However, since I began Buteyko, I am able to breathe wonderfully easily through both nostrils. Prior to Buteyko, I had not breathed through my nose for 12 years. For me, Buteyko means breathing easily through the nose with consequently vastly reduced symptoms.' Dennis

References

Champagne M. Upper airway compromise (UAC) and the long face syndrome. Journal of General Orthodontia. Vol 2. Sept 1991. pp18-25

Coope R. Diseases of the Chest. Livingstone. Edinburgh. 1948. p2

Cottle MH. The work, ways, positions and patterns of nasal breathing (relevance in heart and lung illness). Proceedings of the America Rhinologic Society. 1972

Coventry J. Periodontal Disease. BMJ. 2000. 321. pp36-39

Davies AM, Koenig JS, Thach BT. Characteristics of upper airway chemoreflex prolonged apnea in human infants. Am Rev Respiratory Dis. 1989. 139. pp668–673

Dawes C. Physiological factors affecting salivary flow rate, oral sugar clearance, and the sensation of dry mouth in man. J. Dent Res 1987. 66. pp648-653

Guyton. AC. Human Physiology and Mechanisms of Disease. W.B. Saunders Co. Philadelphia. 1982. pp300, 500-501, 624

Hough A. Physiotherapy in Respiratory Care. Stanley Thornes Ltd. London . 1997. pp27, 28

Magarian GJ. Hyperventilation Syndromes: Infrequently Recognized Common Expressions of Anxiety and Stress. Medicine. The Williams and Wilkins Co. 1982. 61. 4. pp219-236

McDerra EJ, Pollard MA, Curzon ME. The dental status of asthmatic British school children. Paediatric Dent 1998. 20. pp281-287

O'Sullivan EA, Curzon MEJ. Drug Treatments for asthma may cause erosive tooth damage. British Medical J 1998. 317. pp317:820

Rubin RM. Mode of respiration and facial growth. Am J. Orthod. Nov 1980. 78(5). pp504-510

Ryberg M, Moller C, Ericson T. Effect of beta 2 adrenoreceptor agonists on saliva proteins and dental caries in asthmatic children. J Dent Res 1987; 66; 1404-1406

Shaw L, al-Dlaigan YH, Smith A. Childhood asthma and dental erosion. ASDC J Dent Child 2000. 67. pp102-106

Wilson John W, Robertson Colin F. Inhaled steroids – too much of a good thing? MJA. 2002. 177(6). pp288-289

Chapter 5

The Buteyko Institute Method

The Buteyko Institute Method (BIM) tackles the problem of dysfunctional breathing in a practical way, which enables people to take better care of their health and to remove the symptoms that the Carbon Dioxide Syndrome causes.

Chronic hyperventilation causes a small but permanent change to the breathing pattern, which will not revert to the old, healthy way unless it is actively reset (Lum 1994). The Buteyko Institute Practitioner aims to normalise the breathing pattern by using BIM. He or she:

- Creates an awareness of the breathing pattern
- Encourages the correct use of medications
- Teaches a series of simple yet effective breathing exercises
- Provides a set of principles regarding food and physical exercise.

When these strategies are adopted, the respiratory centre begins to accept a more suitable pressure of carbon dioxide and simultaneously a more satisfactory breathing pattern. When this happens the body works more efficiently and symptoms start to disappear. The need for medication is reduced and the person's quality of life improves (Bowler 1998).

Candidates for Buteyko

'The Buteyko Breathing Method is magic. I had tried many cures before Buteyko. None worked long term. Buteyko has relieved all symptoms of asthma. I am still an asthmatic but you wouldn't know it.' Noel

Virtually anyone from four years old can use BIM for improved health and it is currently used for the treatment of asthma, emphysema, snoring, sleep apnoea, allergies, chronic bronchitis, hyperventilation syndrome, chronic fatigue, Raynaud's disease, panic attacks, bronchiectasis, hay fever and chronic sinusitis. Using Buteyko to enhance performance at sports is also becoming increasingly popular and it has been used with some success for the treatment of hypertension, arthritis, epilepsy, cystic fibrosis and diabetes.

While the results of Buteyko often seem magical it is not a magic cure, but the drugs used to treat these conditions are not cures either and Buteyko has the value of no side effects. It works because the respiratory centre is adaptable and can be retrained to accept a more orthodox carbon dioxide pressure (Grippi 1995),which means that the symptoms of chronic hyperventilation are lessened or removed entirely. To read personal stories from people who have learned the Buteyko Method go to Chapter 20.

Buteyko is Not a Quick Fix

Carbon dioxide is so powerful that it has been called the 'hormone of all hormones' and the 'vitamin of all vitamins', and it plays a part in the regulation of every metabolic process in the whole body. Therefore, changes to the breathing pattern cannot be rushed because this affects every cell and the entire body's chemistry and function. For people with certain health problems such as diabetes, the changes must be extra slow, which is why learning Buteyko from a reliable source with a slow and careful approach is a must.

Adults and children learn different Buteyko exercises to change their breathing pattern. Initially the adult exercises take a considerable amount of time but once they are mastered, it is possible to practise them while doing other things, and once breathing patterns have changed then little effort is needed to stay in control. The Buteyko exercises for children on the other hand, take little time and are easy to do. This suits a child's temperament far better than attempting the adult exercises.

Origins of the Buteyko Method

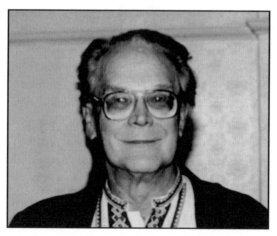

Figure 5:1. Konstantin Pavlovich Buteyko. December 2000.

BIM is named after a Russian doctor, Konstantin Pavlovich Buteyko who was born in Ivanitsa, Ukraine, on 27th January

1923. Buteyko's interest in breathing began while he was enrolled at Medical School in Moscow. He observed that those who are either ill or in pain breathe more than a healthy person. In his third year at medical school Buteyko spent hundreds of hours sitting beside patients' bedsides and noticed that their breathing deepened considerably as they came close to death.

By asking patients to hyperventilate deliberately, Buteyko found that they experienced a wide variety of symptoms, which included fainting. This he was told was due to excessive oxygen reaching the brain, but while doing research Buteyko realised that common thinking on breathing was incorrect because the brain receives less oxygen when you hyperventilate, rather than more. Buteyko also found that the bizarre range of symptoms he had associated with hyperventilation had been documented over eighty years prior to his interest.

During the American Civil War in 1871, a physician called Da Costa first recorded that soldiers were suffering from varied, non-organic symptoms which were originally called 'Soldier's Heart' and 'Da Costa's Syndrome'. Over the years, this chronic hyperventilation has also been called by other names, including: effort syndrome, neurasthenia, cardiac neurosis, neurocirculatory asthenia, hyperventilation syndrome and simply 'stress'. What Buteyko did not find, however, was where anyone had tried to reverse the breathing pattern to see if they could make these symptoms disappear.

Buteyko himself suffered from high blood pressure, a rapid heartbeat and frequent headaches at this time. On checking his own breathing, he found that he was also breathing deeper than is considered normal, so he began experimenting. He found that his symptoms disappeared when he breathed less and returned when he deepened his breathing. From his previous studies he had learned:

- Breathing more than is required for metabolism causes hypocapnia, or low carbon dioxide pressure in the bloodstream.
- Hypocapnia causes smooth muscle spasm and there is smooth muscle wrapped around all hollow parts of the body.
- Hypocapnia agitates the nervous system causing a variety of responses.
- Hypocapnia results in less oxygen released to tissue cells (Bohr effect).
- The brain is especially vulnerable to less oxygen when carbon dioxide pressure is low.

And he apparently now began to speculate that:

- Some diseases are the result of, or are aggravated by breathing too much.
- By voluntarily reducing the amount of air people breathe, symptoms would diminish and good health should be restored.
- Some diseases are not actually diseases at all, but a symptom of, or a defence mechanism against breathing excessively.

He knew that the smallest activity of simply being alive produces carbon dioxide, and once the respiratory centre has accepted a low pressure as normal, then the person will breathe deeper or faster in order to maintain this tension. Buteyko theorised that the opposite would also be true: once the brain adjusted to a higher pressure of carbon dioxide, it would automatically reduce the breathing pattern. By voluntarily reducing the amount of air you breathe for short periods of time, you accustom the respiratory centre to a slightly higher pressure. Buteyko called this process the 'volitional liquidation of deep breathing' or 'volitional breathing normalisation'.

The Disease of Deep Breathing

According to Buteyko (1994), deep breathing is a disease with the potential to exhibit a vast number of symptoms, as is demonstrated in Figure 5.2.

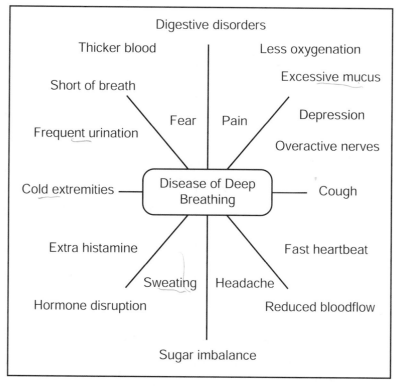

Figure 5:2. Common symptoms caused or exacerbated by the Disease of Deep Breathing.

The symptoms vary, according to your genetic make up and social conditioning factors, which means that both nature and nurture decide how the disease of deep breathing will progress. For example, perhaps a person is born with extra-sensitive nasal passages and unwisely chooses to be a carpenter. Sawdust makes the person sneeze a little at the best of times, but when they hyperventilate, extra sawdust is inhaled and the already sensitive nose reacts violently. The person is now labelled as suffering from rhinitis, rather than breathing too much (Figure 5.3).

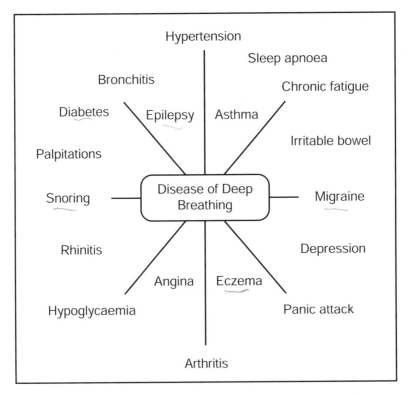

Figure 5:3. The disease of deep breathing is identified as other diseases or conditions.

The idea that deep breathing or hyperventilation is mistaken for other diseases is not confined to the Buteyko viewpoint. The following authors are a small representation of the doctors and researchers who have written about this problem: Fried (1993), Gardner (1996), Gardner and Bass (1989), Lum (1975 and 1978), Magarian (1982), Perera (1988) and Vansteenkiste (1991).

The types of conditions that hyperventilation has been mistaken for include angina, asthma, epilepsy, depression, heart disease, brain tumour, emphysema, acute rheumatic fever, poliomyelitis, peptic ulcer, hypothyroidism, hyperthyroidism, allergies, arthritis, fibrosis and 'nerves'.

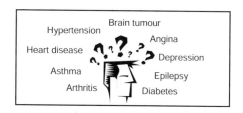

Once the symptoms are manifested, the fact that the breathing pattern is not normal is either still not noticed or it is considered unimportant, because breathing rises when a person is sick. As treatment for the condition begins, the disease of deep breathing gets worse because drugs simply mask the symptoms. This allows the underlying cause hyperventilation to continue unheeded and further symptoms develop as tissue becomes aged and damaged earlier than necessary. Sometimes these symptoms overlap and people receive more than one label as is shown in Figure 5.4.

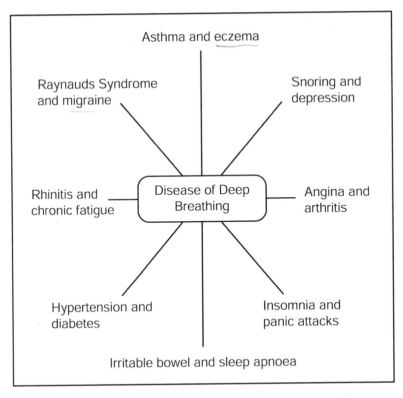

Asthma and eczema

Raynauds Syndrome and migraine

Snoring and depression

Rhinitis and chronic fatigue — Disease of Deep Breathing — Angina and arthritis

Hypertension and diabetes

Insomnia and panic attacks

Irritable bowel and sleep apnoea

Figure 5:4. The Disease of Deep Breathing has a wide range of symptoms that are seemingly unrelated and so the person is frequently diagnosed with more than one condition.

Hidden Hyperventilation

When Buteyko realised that people are largely not aware of their dysfunctional breathing and others seldom notice it either, he coined the term 'hidden hyperventilation' to describe what is commonly known today as chronic hyperventilation or Chronic Hyperventilation Syndrome. We have renamed this problem the Carbon Dioxide Syndrome because the greatest effect of hyperventilation is on the pressure of carbon dioxide, and it is

74

the lack of this gas that largely causes the symptoms. The brain's adaptation to lowered carbon dioxide pressure then perpetuates the syndrome by allowing constant hidden hyperventilation.

Change is Slow in the Field of Medicine

Doctors are trained to look at medicine empirically, with results of controlled tests laid out before them in order to accept new treatments, but sometimes their all too common lack of desire to even consider harmless treatments is hard to comprehend. Examples from history show how unwise this prejudice can be. Ignaz Semmelweiss (1818 -1865) and Joseph Lister (1827 – 1912) were two doctors who were either ignored or considered to be lunatics by their peers for suggesting that doctors should wash their hands before examining patients. Semmelweiss had the idea first and was so bitterly ridiculed that he became deranged and died in a mental institution. Lister was also treated with both indifference and hostility for a number of years before hand washing and sterilisation of instruments finally became common practice.

Buteyko's theory was considered radical and he found little support from his teachers and peers, yet he was fortunately able to continue with his research at a state-funded laboratory for a time. After some years this funding was removed and he was effectively unemployed for most of his adult life, which is a great rarity in a communist country, especially for a well-educated doctor. It is believed that this was largely due to the Russian medical fraternity's inability to accept his theory that hyperventilation is the root cause of many health problems. While he did not suffer like Semmelweiss, Buteyko's life was not easy and if he had not been determined to help mankind there is little doubt that his method would have died out long ago. In 1981, approximately thirty years after his initial discovery, this harmless yet effective means of controlling hyperventilation was finally accepted by the Soviet Health Department and his techniques were finally taught officially in hospitals throughout the USSR.

Development of the Buteyko Method

As the Buteyko Method became more widely used in the treatment of different health problems, the techniques evolved into what they are today. There are a number of techniques and ideas taught as part of the Buteyko Institute Method and some are listed below. It is worth being aware however, that by changing the breathing pattern incorrectly it is possible to both increase the severity of symptoms or to make others appear, which makes learning the Method from a reliable source very important.

Control Pause

The Control Pause is used in conjunction with the pulse to measure the person's health, breathing pattern and likelihood of experiencing symptoms. It is considered healthy for a person to have a Control Pause of at least 40 seconds. To check your own Control Pause get a watch or clock with a second hand and sit in a straight backed chair in sight of the clock face. Breathe normally for two or three minutes. Take note of the depth and speed of your breathing while you wait because you will want to breathe in the same manner once you have finished the pause. After a normal breath out, gently hold the end of your nose with one hand so that you close your nostrils and pause the breathing until you feel the first urge to breathe in again. You time how many seconds you are comfortable holding the nose before needing to inhale again and this length of time is your Control Pause.

As soon as you note the first urge to breathe, take your hand away and breathe normally through your nose. The breathing that you do after the pause should be exactly the same as it was before you began holding your nose.

If your Control Pause time is less than 20 seconds then you probably ticked many of the symptoms in the Hyperventilation Test in chapter three.

Maximum Pause

Sometimes a great emphasis is put on an exercise called the Maximum Pause, which involves holding the breath for as long as you feel you are able to while still being able to breathe through the nose at the end. This could be by the teacher or by the person learning the Method because it seems a fast way to get results since you can really notice something happening.

As the Method has developed over the years, people teaching BIM have placed less emphasis on the Maximum Pause, suggesting that it be used strictly for emergencies and only if instruction has been given by your practitioner, because a sudden boost in carbon dioxide stimulates breathing and causes rapid changes throughout the body. The maximum pause is definitely not the kind of thing that should be used as a party trick.

Extended Pause

The Extended Pause lies between the Control Pause and Maximum Pause. Like the Maximum Pause it has less importance than the rest of the exercises, and while it can be of use to overcome chest tightness for example, it may also cause any number of reactions that are not desired.

Mini Pause

When a person senses that they are getting sick, the Mini Pause is a useful tool to have because hyperventilation can suppress the immune system and by regularly practising this tiny pause the opposite happens; a stimulation of the immune response is created. The person makes the smallest pause in the breathing after a normal exhalation, holding for *no more* than three or four seconds before breathing in normally again. This is repeated every few minutes throughout the day until the sense of impending illness has disappeared.

Nose Clearing Exercise

Possibly the most useful of all the Buteyko exercises for everyday use when first learning Buteyko, is the nose clearing exercise. This exercise can be performed while sitting, standing or walking. It basically includes holding the breath in a similar way to the Control Pause but either nodding the head or walking around and maintaining strict and careful nose breathing at the finish. It can be used whenever the nose is blocked and also several times consecutively in a short time. It is described more fully in Chapter Four.

Shallow or Reduced Breathing

When the Buteyko Method was first taken outside of Russia to Australia, the main Buteyko exercise for adults was called 'Shallow Breathing'. This was a direct translation from the Russian language to English. However, 'shallow' breathing in English is commonly thought of as being rapid, upper chest breathing and is one way of hyperventilating – the very thing that you are trying to avoid.

People were constantly making mistakes with the exercise, so people teaching BIM renamed the exercise as 'Reduced Breathing' because this is actually what you are attempting to do when you practise this exercise, so it seems more appropriate.

Horse Rider

To assist a person to reduce their breathing, the horse rider position may be implemented. As the name implies, this exercise requires a person to sit as though riding a horse: knees apart with thighs sloping towards the floor, abdomen lengthened so that the back is straight and shoulders very relaxed. Diaphragmatic breathing becomes easy to do when sitting like this and there should be little or no upper chest movement.

Anti-Hyperventilation Exercises

Hyperventilation attacks are notoriously hard to stop by conventional means but the BIM includes a number of exercises that are used to interrupt acute hyperventilation and prevent hyperventilation attacks from continuing.

The BIM uses a combination of these exercises along with some others and a few points regarding lifestyle to assist the person with hidden hyperventilation to restore normal breathing patterns. As breathing returns to normal then the need for the exercises also diminishes.

The Buteyko Institute of Breathing and Health

The Buteyko Method came to Australia in 1990 via Russian practitioner Alexander Stalmatski. Australia was the first country outside of the Soviet Bloc to have sufficient teachers for local Asthma Foundations and medical practitioners to take note of 'Buteyko', as it commonly became known there. Within four years, practitioners decided to form a body that would make Buteyko practitioners accountable to both the Method and to the people they teach. It was hoped that by having a self-regulating body Buteyko would quickly gain credibility, and so the Buteyko Institute of Breathing and Health Inc. (BIBH) was formed. Today it is an international body with members in many different countries.

The BIBH has a number of basic functions. Two of the most important are regulation of the way that the Method is taught and the way that new Practitioners are trained. These are included because it is easy to confuse Buteyko and other modalities of treatment. When commencing a Buteyko course, attendees begin to practise breathing exercises to improve their health. If they also began taking vitamins at the same time, they would not be sure exactly what was making them feel better. If the Buteyko Practitioner had provided the vitamins as well as the breathing exercises then it would be even more confusing, and quite likely that the vitamins would get the credit. This is likely for two reasons:

- Many people have been conditioned to believe that there is a 'pill for every ill'.
- Many people incorrectly assume that nothing can be wrong with their breathing.

80

The BIBH reminds its practitioner members that the Method is almost entirely about teaching people to breathe properly, while also incorporating some ideas on diet, physical exercise and sleep patterns that assist in the reduction of stress.

While Professor Buteyko was alive he was the patron of the BIBH and together with his wife and her son, conducted training with several members. He did not live long enough to see his Method incorporated into the health systems of countries other than his own, as he died May 2nd, 2003. To read about some of the Buteyko Institute Practitioners turn to Chapter Twenty.

References

Bowler SD. et al. Buteyko breathing techniques in asthma: a blinded randomised controlled trial. MJA 1998. 169. pp575-578

Buteyko KP. Buteiko's Method. Method of Volitional Control of Deep Breathing. Guide for training. Voskresensk. 1994

Fried R. The Psychology and Physiology of Breathing. Plenum Press. New York 1993. pp195-196

Gardner WN. The Pathophysiology of Hyperventilation Disorders. Chest. 1996. 109. pp516-534

Gardner WN, Bass C. Hyperventilation in clinical practice. British J Hospital Medicine. 1989. 41. pp73-81

Grippi M. Pulmonary Pathophysiology. J.B. Lippincott Company. Philadelphia. 1995. p249

Lum LC. Behavioural and Psychological Approaches to Breathing Disorders. Ed. B.H. Timmons & R Ley. Plenum. New York. 1994. p116

Lum LC. Hyperventilation: The tip and the iceberg. J Psychosom Res. 1975. 19. pp375-383

Lum, L.C. Respiratory Alkalosis and Hypocarbia The role of carbon dioxide in the body economy. Chest, Heart and Stroke Journal. 1978. 3(4). pp31-34

Magarian GJ. Hyperventilation Syndromes: Infrequently Recognized Common Expressions of Anxiety and Stress. Medicine. The Williams and Wilkins Co. 1982. 61 (4). pp219-236

Perera J. The Hazards of heavy breathing. New Scientist, Dec 1988:46-48.

Vansteenkiste J, Rochette F, Demedts M. Diagnostic tests of hyperventilation syndrome. European Respir J. 1991. 4. pp393-399

Chapter 6

Asthma

Asthma is a strange condition — there is a sensation of not having enough air, yet the more you breathe, the worse it gets! This is unusual because when feeling hungry for example, once you eat the sensation is gone. It is perfectly logical, however, when asthma is considered from the Buteyko point of view. If hyperventilation is too severe or chronic, the entire body is in danger from loss of carbon dioxide and so airways close to prevent this. Resisting this defence mechanism by struggling to breathe more air only makes them close more tightly.

In spite of all the research into asthma, it is on the increase and is the only treatable life-threatening condition in the western world with a rising death rate, with up to 86% of deaths being preventable (Grampian study 1994). English-speaking countries have the highest incidence (Holt 2000), and the incidence of asthma in these countries has practically doubled over the past twenty years (Holgate 1998). Perhaps this is due to better diagnosis, but it has also been suggested that today homes are too clean. With fewer children in a household, less dust and dirt and less exposure to infections and parasites, it is believed that the immune system is being reprogrammed. This theory also implies that non-English speaking western countries are less clean, which fortunately makes this hypothesis less likely to be supported internationally. The view of Buteyko Practitioners is that the change in lifestyle has created a growing problem of dysfunctional breathing, which is commonly labelled 'asthma'.

Asthma is described by the acronym R.O.A.D. – Reversible Obstructive Airway Disorder and is defined by Asher (1987) and others, as having three components:

1. Spasm of smooth muscles wrapped around the airways.
2. Increased mucus production.
3. Inflammation of the inner airway walls.

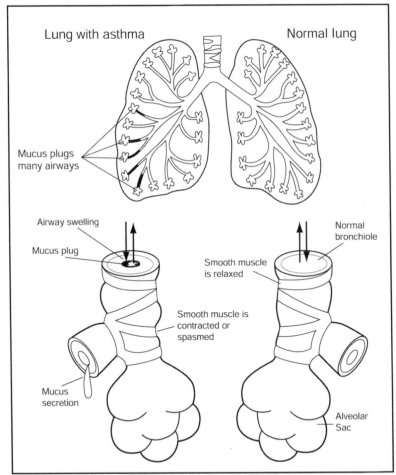

Figure 6:1. Comparison of the asthmatic and the normal lung.

Asthma Differences

A person who does not have asthma often assumes that asthma is all the same – wheezing, coughing and experiencing shortness of breath. In fact, the way that asthma presents itself differs from person to person by a number of factors. These differences include:

- Asthma symptoms
- The age that asthma first appears
- The things that trigger an attack
- Severity of the attacks
- Treatments to control the symptoms.

Symptoms
Common asthma symptoms include:

- Chest tightness
- Wheezing
- Coughing
- Shortness of breath.

People with asthma may have some or all of these symptoms, while others just quietly go blue. The symptoms can change, perhaps wheezing one day and coughing the next. It is often believed that wheezing is the main symptom of asthma, but this is not necessarily correct because other conditions can also make a person wheeze – bronchitis or having a heavy cold, for example. When smooth muscle spasm, inflammation and mucus production are extreme, airways can become plugged with mucus and air does not reach the alveoli in that part of the lung, causing the section to collapse. When many airways are plugged, gas exchange is seriously impaired and breathing may be so weak that it is impossible to wheeze. While there is no evidence of wheezing, medical help is badly needed.

Age

The age that a person first gets asthma can range from early childhood to senior adults. One possible reason for this is that the immune system changes with age. A baby and tiny child's immune system relies largely on being able to vomit at the least provocation and having copious amounts of mucus. These two components help to keep unwanted substances out of the body, but a child with tiny airways and lots of mucus will wheeze and cough, which could easily be mistaken for asthma. Once the wheezy baby's airways grow larger and the immune system places less reliance on mucus production, symptoms can drop dramatically and by the time the child is eight years old, the lungs, airways and alveoli have grown so much that there is ten times more space for gas exchange than there is in a newborn baby (Haas 1987).

Allergens are potentially harmful foreign bodies that are touched, eaten or inhaled. The immune system responds in a number of ways to keep them out of the body, destroy, or to contain them in one place by creating inflammation, heat or antibodies. While this is a useful mechanism to prevent infection or poisoning, the response itself can be troublesome. For example, cat dander (tiny scales of fur) is not poisonous, yet antibodies can cause such a strong reaction to dander that the reaction makes the person extremely sick.

IgE is an antibody that is found in the skin, digestive tract and airways. Babies and young children have lots of IgE reactions to foods. By the time the child is ten years old this has largely disappeared, however the IgE reaction to inhaled substances increases. By age of thirty, the IgE antibody has begun to subside and the allergies it has caused have dropped considerably. The belief that people 'grow out' of asthma in a seven-year cycle could have come about because of these changes to the body. In fact, only 5% of people who have chronic asthma as children remain symptom-free as adults (Asher 1987, Haas 1987). A person who is predisposed by genetics to asthma may get it later in life as a response to a lifetime of stress, and the 'wear and tear' that this causes reveals itself in the lungs.

Triggers

An asthma attack can be triggered by almost anything. Triggers change not only from person to person, but also within the same person, for example today it could be eating chocolate and tomorrow it could be exercise. The most common asthma provocations are:

- Physical activities – exercise, exertion, running, playing sport, having sex, doing housework.
- Illness, especially chest infections, colds or the flu.
- Seasonal or weather types and changes - wind, humidity and cold weather being the worst offenders.
- Sudden temperature change – especially warm to cold.
- Sleeping.
- Foods and drinks. These vary enormously from person to person but the main culprits appear to be: very cold food or drinks (like ice cream and beer); chocolate; dairy products; chicken soup; honey; fish or shellfish; strawberries; nuts; caffeine-type drinks; alcohol.
- Strong odours or perfumes.
- Household cleaners.
- Aerosol sprays.
- Using a peak flow meter (device to check asthmatic condition).

- Pollen, grasses, flowers.
- Exposure to animals such as cats, dogs, horses or birds.
- Emotions – excitement, anticipation, worry, stress, laughter or tears.
- Smoke, fumes.
- Gastric reflux.

Once a trigger has set off the asthma symptoms, the person instinctively breathes harder to cope with the airway restriction. If particular attention is paid to the breathing before the symptoms occur, it is noticed that the person is already breathing more than usual. (Groen 1979, Hibbert 1988, McFadden 1968). This is because triggers act like a stress on the body, boosting breathing and in turn creating the symptoms.

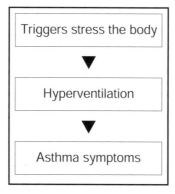

Figure 6:2. Triggers create a stress, which starts the asthma cycle.

This becomes more obvious when you consider that laughing and blowing into a peak flow meter, both of which increase the breathing pattern dramatically, are common asthma triggers (Anderson Price 1992, Lim 1989). Even in an allergy-type attack caused by pollen, the breathing increases as part of the alarm reaction. To a person with asthma, it becomes patently obvious that it is necessary to breathe more than usual to create the symptoms. It may even be noticed that the more air breathed, the more symptoms appear, as was documented by Hibbert and Pilsbury in their 1998 study entitled 'Demonstration and treatment of hyperventilation causing asthma.'

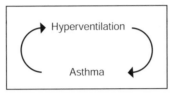

Figure 6:3. Hyperventilation and asthma are intertwined.

People with asthma often spend a lot of time and energy either eliminating triggers or avoiding their triggers, but while nothing is done about hyperventilation it simply gets worse. At the onset of asthma, perhaps only cats and exercise were triggers, but after a time it seems that virtually everything on the planet sets it off, even though the person owns a better vacuum cleaner, no longer has a cat, stays away from smoky bars and goes for a walk instead of a run.

Asthma Severity

For people with mild to moderate asthma, the attacks ordinarily occur between two and four times a month and they are easily dealt with by taking a puff of reliever medication. The incidents are not life threatening and are generally thought of as a nuisance. As asthma becomes severe, episodes occur with greater frequency and strength and even the thought of asthma becomes threatening. Preventive medication is taken to lessen the severity and frequency of these attacks. People with chronic asthma find that the asthma-free periods get shorter until the symptoms are present nearly all the time and asthma now dominates their life.

Severity can be trigger-related. For example, in spring when the pollen count is up, asthma might take a turn for the worse, but by summer it has improved again. The severity of asthma can also change over a period of time. Perhaps asthma starts with mild attacks but it gradually becomes more severe and instead of only taking a reliever, preventive medication is required as well, or instead of never needing oral steroids, they are necessary once or twice a year.

Asthma Treatments

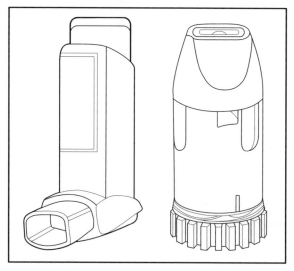

Figure 6:4. Typical styles of inhalers.

Even though there are several different brands and delivery systems of medication, conventional asthma treatment has changed little over the past forty years. There are two basic types of drugs – relievers and preventers. Relievers act on nerves in the airway smooth muscle, relaxing them or preventing the muscle spasm. Their use is currently recommended only to be taken 'as needed' to treat asthma symptoms when they appear.

Each dose is effective for three to four hours. Preventers reduce or prevent inflammation and lessen the reaction to allergens. The purpose of taking a preventer is to lessen the need for relievers and they are taken regularly whether the person has asthma symptoms or not. When the symptoms of asthma are worse, all medication is stepped up and when the symptoms ease, it is stepped down again.

Buteyko is not about throwing drugs away. It is about using them correctly and fortunately as symptoms drop quickly when you apply the Buteyko Method, so does the need for medication.

Reliever Medication

In 1976 there was a sudden increase in the number of deaths from asthma in New Zealand, and until 1989 it had the highest death rate from asthma in the world. This was attributed to the use of a reliever drug called Fenoterol (Holt 2000) and led to a large number of studies worldwide into the safety and efficacy of reliever medications as a whole. These studies overwhelmingly showed that the overuse of reliever medication can worsen asthma (Crane 1993, Inman 1969, Speizer 1968). This could be for a number of reasons:

- Nerve endings that stimulate the relaxation of smooth muscle tend to disappear with the overuse of relievers (Schuster 1991). This leads to 'floppy airways' where mild triggers cause the airways to narrow or collapse.
- Inhaled irritants scar the airway walls. Damaged airways do not work as effectively as healthy ones (Hough 1997). Airways close to prevent the inhalation of these substances. Taking relievers causes the airways to remain open and irritants may be inhaled more deeply, causing extensive damage.

- Relievers stimulate breathing (Ameisen 1997). When taken repeatedly, the brain becomes used to a lower pressure of carbon dioxide and maintains a heightened breathing pattern with less oxygen released to tissues. The more air breathed, the more breathless the person becomes and the more irritants inhaled.

- Taking relievers regularly can lead to their overdose, which alone can be harmful, but it can also lead to neglect of preventer medications because relievers may mask symptoms. By doing this, the severity of the situation is not immediately recognised and it could mean that inflammation is rampant before action is taken (Anderson Price 1992).

Currently most national asthma guidelines recommend relievers to be used only as required and no more than twice a week (Milne 1996). If relievers are required more frequently, then it is recommended that preventer medication be adjusted (National Asthma Education Programme 1991). But the guidelines were not like this prior to 1990. In those days it was common for asthmatics to take relievers as often as they wanted and to use them in a preventer-type role, i.e. reliever was taken before activities that commonly caused symptoms, such as before playing sport, going for a walk, sleeping or visiting a friend with a cat. In addition, many doctors prescribed relievers on a regular daily schedule (e.g. three times a day), in the mistaken belief that it would improve overall asthma control (Guidelines for the Diagnostics and Management of Asthma 1997). When relievers are used like this, the asthmatic condition can deteriorate rapidly and the death rate rises dramatically (Jackson 1982, Sears 1990). When current asthma management guidelines of using relievers only as needed, and altering preventive medication when relievers are needed more than twice a week are applied, the death rate from asthma drops considerably (Neville 1991).

Even with this knowledge freely available to people with asthma, it is ironic that the medication that appears to do the most harm is the same medication that is most popular. People have no qualms about taking their reliever medication because they cannot see their changing airways and even if they could, a person will do anything to breathe! The reliever medication is seen as their friend, their 'little blue mate', because it takes the symptoms away – in the short term.

Preventer Medication

Preventer medications on the other hand, particularly the steroid types, are often considered the enemy because everyone has heard about steroids and their side effects. Not only do these medications cause side effects, but also they are most obvious (Hough 1997). People see the bruising, hear the husky voice and notice the high incidence of oral thrush and chest infections. They hear about cataracts, osteoporosis and Cushing's syndrome, but what people do not realise is that their 'little blue mate' could be making their asthma worse and consequently increasing preventer use in the long-term.

Corticosteroids stabilise and restore the nerve endings that stimulate the opening of airways and so are likely to improve their tone and efficiency (Brisco 1997, Cochrane 1987). When taken regularly, inhaled corticosteroids moderate the frequency and severity of asthma symptoms (Juniper 1990, Sears 1992). In fact there is ten times less risk of fatal or near-fatal asthma attacks when these drugs are taken, compared to using relievers only (Brisco 1997). It is therefore infinitely preferable to take a small amount of steroid medication than a lot of reliever. The chances of dying from uncontrolled asthma are MUCH greater than dying of osteoporosis.

Controller Medication

'Controllers' are similar to relievers except that they are stronger and open the airways for a much longer period - as long as twelve to fifteen hours. As a comparison of strength, it is estimated that taking one fifty-microgram puff of Salmeterol (controller) is equivalent to taking five puffs of Salbutamol (reliever) every four to six hours (Smyth 1993). It is therefore not surprising that studies showing a worsening of the asthmatic condition have already begun to surface since these drugs have become more widely used (Crane 1993, Downes 1995).

Controllers are usually prescribed once or twice a day and can take up to thirty minutes to take effect. Because of this time delay it is possible for the person to panic when they do not get immediate relief and take more than the recommended dose, so they should never be used to treat an acute asthma attack (Adams 1998, Guidelines for the Diagnostics and Management of Asthma 1997).

The main fear however, with people taking controllers is that they could mask asthma symptoms and people become less aware that their condition is deteriorating (McIvor 1998). For example, an asthmatic might have an allergic reaction to cats and so every effort is made to avoid them. Taking controller medications will keep the airway smooth muscle relaxed, moderating the symptoms, so that there is less awareness of inhaling the dander. In the background however, the immune system is working hard to keep it out, or at best, to contain the dander in one place. Controllers do not stop the inflammation and mucus production caused by exposure to the cat dander. In fact, the widened airways will allow further penetration of the dander, causing the immune system to put up an even greater response, which could lead to a severe attack a short while later. In a British study, it was found that the risk of dying from taking Salmeterol was three times greater than from taking Salbutamol (Castle 1993).

Combination Controller – Preventer Medications

The latest trend in asthma medications is to combine controller type medications and steroid preventers into one delivery device. The fear that asthmatics will take reliever medications regularly without taking a steroid preventer is overcome by combining the two drugs into one inhaler. The long-term effect of taking a strong reliever twice a day instead of no more than the recommended twice a week, even when combined with a steroid, will no doubt be revealed in the near future.

WARNING: While drug therapy is not a perfect way to control asthma, for most people it is the only way that they have and potentially life-saving medication should not be discarded. Taking a puff of reliever can stop an attack from getting worse and in some instances the discontinuation of steroid medications can be fatal. Therefore consultation with your doctor is a MUST before any medication is changed or discarded.

Other Treatments and Remedies

In addition to drug therapies, other treatments of asthma include:

- Desensitisation, a treatment that involves taking a small amount of the suspected irritant regularly, in the hope that the immune system will stop reacting to it.
- Osteopathy.
- Chiropractics.
- Herbal treatments.
- Eating of various special foods, vitamins or minerals, such as the omega three fish oils.

- Relaxation techniques such as yoga or tai chi.
- Physiotherapy breathing techniques.
- Swimming or other regular forms of exercise.

To someone who does not have asthma, it is impossible to imagine how frightening it is to not easily breathe. The panic that can accompany asthma is one reason why it is sometimes thought that asthma is 'all in the mind'. The fact that worldwide, thousands of people die from asthma every year does little to change this misconception. In an effort to eliminate or diminish the symptoms, people with asthma either give up activities or take action in an attempt to stop the symptoms from occurring. These things often include altering the diet; taking vitamins; exercising regularly or less vigorously; doing meticulous housework but no longer using aerosols or pungent cleaners; avoiding cigarette smoke and perfumes; getting rid of pets, and in extreme cases even moving house or country. While the person quite rightly does any possible thing in order to breathe easily, at the same time, their world is getting smaller and smaller in the attempt to control asthma. What is actually happening in this situation, is instead of the person controlling their asthma, the asthma is controlling the person.

The Hyperventilation - Asthma Connection

Conventional medicine recognises that people with asthma hyperventilate (Anderson Price 1992) but it is usually thought to occur only after the airways become constricted. This is because breathing is very noticeable during an attack, usually in excess of twenty-five breaths per minute and the strong accessory muscles of the upper chest are used to breathe with instead of the diaphragm (Hough 1997). Buteyko Practitioners acknowledge this, but also recognise that hyperventilation occurs before the symptoms appear. Breathing between ten and fourteen litres of air a minute when no symptoms are present is commonly noted in asthma studies (Bowler 1998, Hibbert 1988).

It is unlikely that anyone has experienced an asthma attack when they are breathing quietly and softly through their nose and the idea that breathing too much will cause breathlessness is not new, nor does it only belong to Buteyko Practitioners. New Zealand physiotherapist Bernice Thompson wrote a book entitled 'Better Breathing', which was published in 1967. She states: "If he is not instructed in relaxed, normal breathing, the 'effort' breather will tend to become more and more breathless as time passes."

Hyperventilation can cause the three aspects of all asthma attacks:

1. Spasm of smooth muscles wrapped around the airways
2. Increased mucus production
3. Inflammation of the inner airway walls.

This is done in a threefold operation - loss of carbon dioxide, increased inhalation of irritants and the cooling and drying of airways (Deal 1979, van Elshout 1991).

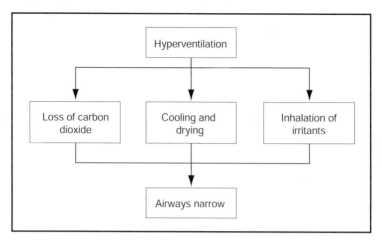

Figure 6:5. Hyperventilation causes asthma.

When carbon dioxide pressure drops or the airways lose heat and water they narrow to prevent further loss (Milne 1996). Airway narrowing protects the body against loss of carbon dioxide, prevents the airways from cooling and drying, and it prevents intrusion of irritants that can damage the airways or make the person ill (Lumb 2000).

A major component of airway narrowing is histamine-related and extra histamine is released when carbon dioxide tension is low (Kontos 1972). Histamine constricts airway smooth muscle, creates inflammation, and both generates and thickens mucus (Fried 1993). Mucus helps to keep the airways clean and moist but an overproduction clogs the airways, preventing irritants from moving further into the body and making it more difficult to breathe. Asthmatics as a whole produce more mucus than other people because their mucus-producing cells are larger and more numerous (Lumb 2000).

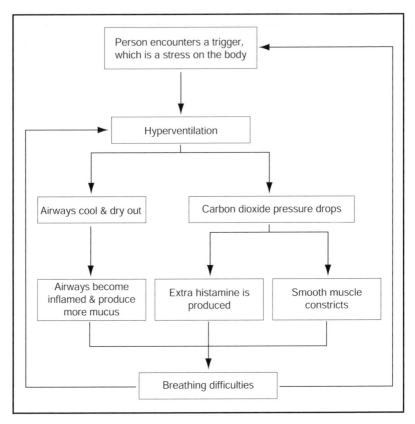

Figure 6:6. The hyperventilation - asthma cycle.

Even without cooling and drying airways or releasing extra histamine, hyperventilation will constrict the airways due to the direct loss of carbon dioxide (Kontos 1972, Van Elshout 1991) and also cause a drop in oxygen reaching tissues, which increases the production of lactic acid. All of these factors stimulate breathing, creating a vicious circle.

The asthma trigger may not involve an irritant; it could be exercising hard that intensifies the breathing pattern. Mucous glands now produce extra mucus to protect the drying airways and as over-breathing continues, it becomes sticky, which often causes coughing. Coughing involves deep breathing and generally worsens asthma symptoms.

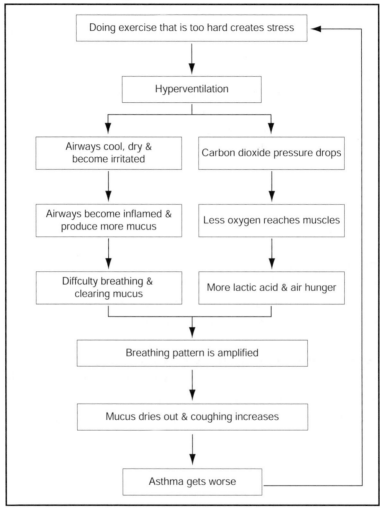

Figure 6:7. Exercise and asthma.

The nervous system is the cornerstone of a person's ability to perceive, adapt to, and interact with the world. It is the means by which people receive, process and then respond to messages from the environment and from inside the body. Part of this system is called the autonomic nervous system (ANS). The autonomic nervous system is divided into two parts: the sympathetic nervous system and the parasympathetic nervous system. Both systems are involved with metabolism and often work in opposition. For example, the sympathetic system is concerned with metabolic processes that use energy. The parasympathetic system is concerned primarily with metabolic processes that conserve energy.

In the airways, stimulation of the parasympathetic system causes bronchial tubes to constrict, whereas stimulating the sympathetic nervous system produces the opposite reaction (dilation). In normal airways, a balance between these two systems maintains comfortable breathing but in asthmatic airways there is sometimes an imbalance favouring the parasympathetic system that produces narrowing or constriction of the airways.

An overactive parasympathetic nervous system, caused by low carbon dioxide tension, could explain why such nonspecific stimuli such as smoke, viruses and even sudden weather changes trigger wheezing in people with both allergic and non-allergic asthma.

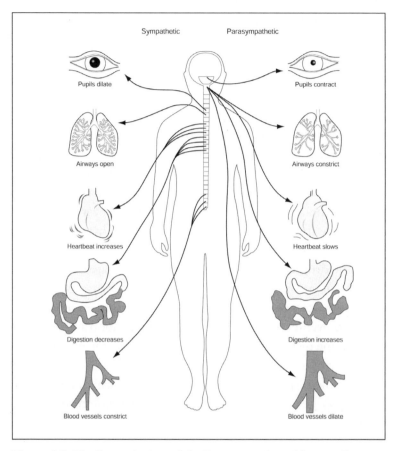

Figure 6:8. The Sympathetic and the Parasympathetic Nervous Systems totally affect the way the body works.

Asthma: A Defence Mechanism

Supporters of the Buteyko theory believe asthma is one of the body's inherent defence mechanisms against hyperventilation and the subsequent loss of carbon dioxide that has a disastrous effect on the health. If a person hyperventilated until carbon dioxide pressure got down so low that the body could not compensate for the Respiratory Alkalosis, death would result. To prevent this from happening, the airways begin to narrow and constrict when the pressure drops too low – McFadden and Lyons (1968) noted airway obstruction when the carbon dioxide pressure was down to 24.6 mm Hg.

By partially closing, the airways prevent further loss of carbon dioxide and allow a slight build-up. During an asthma attack it is considerably harder to breathe out than it is to breathe in, which supports this theory, as it appears that the body is trying to retain the air inside the lungs. Taking reliever medication to override this natural defence means that if hyperventilation continues unchecked, more carbon dioxide will be lost and when the drug wears off, the airways will close again. It is likely that this is a major factor as to why the overuse of reliever medication can considerably worsen the asthmatic condition. Steroid preventer medication reduces inflammation and dampens the immune response to allergens, which is helpful in controlling asthma symptoms. However at the same time it also suppresses the immune response to bacteria and viruses which means that the person gets sick more often, which is a common asthma trigger.

WARNING: This is NOT a recommendation for anyone to stop taking medication because asthma can kill. Being sensible, using medication correctly and seeking timely medical help will prevent this. When you apply the Buteyko Method there is a huge reduction in the need for this defence mechanism. However, it is important to keep your asthma inhaler handy and use it if you need to – one or two puffs of reliever can stop a bad attack from becoming severe. It is only the *overuse* of relievers that should be avoided (Crane 1989).

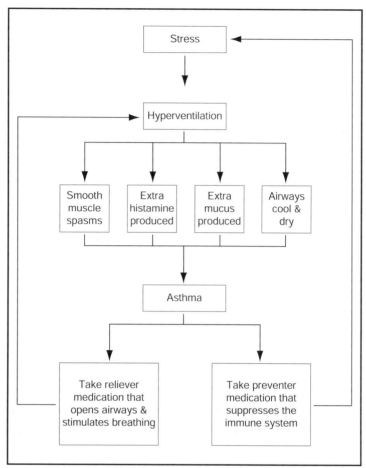

Figure 6:9. The asthma-medication connection.

Airways Can Stay Closed Even as Carbon Dioxide Increases

Before an asthma attack starts and during the early stages, it is likely that oxygen pressure is normal and carbon dioxide is low in the bloodstream (McFadden 1968), but this changes as airways swell, smooth muscles spasm and thick mucus plugs airways.

If the plugging becomes severe and more airways are literally sealed up, then less gas exchange can take place and the work of breathing becomes much greater than normal. Under normal resting conditions approximately 5% of the oxygen we inhale is used for fuel to breathe with, but when the lungs are obstructed this may increase to about 25% (Price Anderson 1992), which means that a lot more carbon dioxide is produced than normal as a result of this extra work. There may also come a point when the plugging is so severe that entire sections of the lungs collapse as they are cut off from ventilation. In this situation, sufficient oxygen cannot get into the bloodstream and carbon dioxide cannot get out. This is the case with 'Status asthmaticus' or extremely severe asthma, which builds over many days with ever-increasing symptoms. This kind of asthma is extremely dangerous and must be treated immediately. Do NOT sit at home waiting to get better.

Extra oxygen, food and water are required when you have asthma because it takes more energy to breathe. However the desire to eat or drink diminishes during an attack, making it easy to become dehydrated and malnourished. After a few days of dehydration and over-breathing, the airways become very dry and mucus is increasingly difficult to shift. As more and more airways become plugged with mucus, it becomes harder for the gas exchange process to take place, and ultimately more sections of the lungs collapse. Even though the circulatory system can make some adjustments for this reduction in gas exchange, there is still some blood flowing past alveoli that is not functioning, which creates a shortfall in oxygen and a build-up of carbon dioxide in the bloodstream.

In the lungs however, carbon dioxide is likely to still be low because of the speed and force that the person is breathing at and this could maintain the spasm of the smooth muscle in the airways. They will not relax until the breathing slows and some normality of pressure in this area is restored, or reliever medications are taken which force their relaxation.

Because of reliever medications, the spasm of the smooth muscle is a relatively easy problem to solve, but the immune and inflammatory responses are more challenging. Successful treatment of severe asthma requires the use of strong and fast-acting corticosteroids to immobilise and reduce the reactions.

The graphs below in Figure 6.10 show that as asthma worsens and the amount of air forcefully breathed out in one second (FEV_1) gets less, the amount of energy it takes to breathe increases, the pH dives and the blood gases become distinctly unhealthy. It is possible that another contributing factor to the success steroids have in reducing asthma symptoms is that they cause a state of metabolic alkalosis (Tortora 1984). To compensate for this the body may reduce the breathing pattern, which begins to eliminate the need for the defence mechanism of airway narrowing. If the state of respiratory acidosis has already been reached due to severe airway plugging, then taking steroids will help to restore normal pH and allow the body to function more normally. At the same time it is reducing inflammation and allergic responses, which causes breathing to become easier as the swelling goes down, and mucus stops clogging the airways.

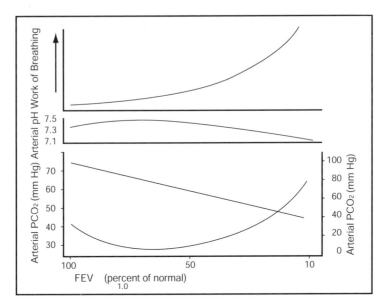

Figure 6:10. The work of breathing. Copied with permission from Pathophysiology. Clinical Concepts of Disease Processes. Price and Wilson. Mosby-Year Book Inc. 1992.

Improve Your Asthma Control

You can help yourself to reduce the incidence of asthma in a number of ways, which include:

- Use preventer medication the way it has been prescribed.
- If more than two puffs of reliever medication are required within one week then seek advice on improving your asthma control.
- If you require reliever medication more than three times in a day then your asthma is completely out of control and you should not delay in getting to a doctor.
- Keep a diary of symptoms, foods that you eat, the

weather, activities and any extraordinary occurrences in your life. This way you may be able to track the worst of your triggers, which may make it possible to eliminate some of them.

- Dust and the dust mite are common triggers and impossible to avoid, but vacuuming regularly, removing dried flowers, stuffed toys and other dust traps from the bedroom and using a damp cloth while dusting may help.
- Do not let pets sleep in the bedroom.
- Maintain a sensible and healthy diet and avoid eating a large meal in the two-hour period before going to sleep.
- Keep as physically fit as you can, but use common sense. This means that if exercise gives you asthma, then cut back a little.
- Breathe through your nose as much as possible.

Buteyko Can Help

'Since learning the Buteyko breathing method, Hannah has seemed fitter and more healthy. She has not visited our GP for over a year now and any asthma problems we have coped with by using the breathing techniques.' Alison (Mother)

Lungs are intended to be sterile, which is why the nose is such an effective filter, and deliberately inhaling substances directly into the lungs is ordinarily considered a bad idea. This is stressed repeatedly in 'Quit Smoking' campaigns, but is seldom, if ever, mentioned to people with regard to asthma medication. Buteyko is not about frightening people regarding their medication, nor is it about throwing drugs away. It is about using medication as recommended by international guidelines. Fortunately as symptoms drop dramatically within a few weeks of starting to use the Buteyko Method, so does the need for reliever medication. This enables the reduction of preventers also within the near future.

Medical studies show that asthmatics regularly breathe more than a healthy person and have low carbon dioxide pressure in the bloodstream, with an average tension of 33 mm Hg not uncommon (Bowler 1998, McFadden 1968). Asthma symptoms begin to occur when the pressure drops to approximately 29 mm Hg or slightly lower in the blood (McFadden 1968). A person with the normal carbon dioxide tension of 40 mm Hg will be able to do more over-breathing before reaching the 29 mm Hg threshold than someone who already has a pressure of 33 mm Hg.

Pressure of carbon dioxide in arterial blood	Litres of air breathed in one minute while resting	Results
40 mm Hg	4 - 6	Normal breathing without constriction
33 mm Hg	10 - 14	Requiring daily medication
29 mm Hg	15 +	Airway constriction

Table 6.1. An asthmatic with low carbon dioxide tension will have more asthma symptoms than a person with normal tension.

Instead of trying to breathe more often and more deeply, the Buteyko Method teaches the asthmatic to automatically breathe less and more slowly, as a healthy person would. This enables the bronchial tubes to relax and relieves asthma symptoms.

The crux of the Buteyko Method is this:

- Healthy people have normal levels of carbon dioxide (40 mm Hg in arterial blood and 46 mm Hg in venal blood) as stated in all medical textbooks.
- Hyperventilation is an abnormality of breathing control and is defined as breathing in excess of metabolic needs. It lowers carbon dioxide and raises the blood pH (Gardner 1995).
- After a period of continual hyperventilation, carbon dioxide tension becomes chronically low and the respiratory centre adapts to this low pressure, automatically increasing the breathing to maintain it (Lum 1994).
- Just as the body adapts to an abnormally low pressure, it is capable of readjusting to the previous healthy pressure (Grippi 1995).
- As the breathing pattern becomes more normal, symptoms subside (Graham 1996)

Since breathing is continuous and automatic, there is no way for individuals to monitor their every breath. The only way to change the breathing pattern is to 'recondition the brain' or teach it to breathe properly again. When following the Buteyko programme, the breathing pattern is deliberately changed for short periods and carbon dioxide pressure is raised slightly. If this is done regularly, the respiratory centre starts to adapt to a slightly higher pressure of carbon dioxide, just like it does every night during sleep. At first it is necessary to complete many sequences of the special exercises and to follow some basic principles so that the brain does not switch back to a lower level shortly afterwards, and once the respiratory centre has adjusted to a healthier carbon dioxide pressure then the asthmatic is able to withstand more trigger-related stress before symptoms appear.

'Who ever thought that breathing (or should I say the lack of it) would so greatly improve asthma to the stage where over the past month I have in total used my Ventolin (including the initial week), 3 times instead of an average of 114 times or more! Wow!' Julie

Testing Buteyko

At the time of writing only a handful of trials have examined the efficacy of the Buteyko Method in the western world. The first trial took place in Brisbane, Australia in 1994 – 1995 with Tess Graham teaching the Buteyko Method. She has kindly lent her findings and thoughts regarding it:

'When the former Buteyko Australia Pty Ltd. and the Australian Association of Asthma Foundations agreed in 1994 to trial the Buteyko Method for asthma, in Brisbane, I was appointed by Buteyko Australia to teach the method to the trial subjects. I saw the clinical trial as a wonderful opportunity to produce scientific evidence that hyperventilation was common to all with asthma, not just a subset, and that Buteyko, by restoring correct breathing, would reduce asthma symptoms and the need for medication in people with asthma. I hoped that this would lead to Buteyko being made known and available to all people with asthma, more Buteyko practitioners would be trained and that we would see an end to the asthma epidemic.

For the clinical trial, I taught the course over 7 days and as I lived over

1000 km from Brisbane, this meant that follow-up consultations had to be by phone. Allowance for this was written into the trial protocol, as it is an essential component of Buteyko training. Many of the trial subjects were severe long-term asthmatics, having had asthma for an average 23 years duration.

The trial was a 'blinded' study. Both groups were learning breathing exercises for asthma. The people I taught were not told that they were learning the Buteyko Method. Another physiotherapist was teaching 'conventional' breathing exercises and management techniques to the Control group in another room on the same floor of the Queensland Asthma Foundation building. An observer commented to me on day four that there was a clearly visible and audible difference in the way the two sets of people were breathing when they got to the top of the stairs.

The Buteyko group achieved overwhelmingly positive results, reducing symptoms by an average 71% and reducing bronchodilator medications by an average of 96% and steroid preventer medication by an average of 49% over three months, while experiencing improved quality of life.

The research was published in the Medical Journal of Australia in December 1998. It was disappointing that the publication of the results did not lead to the acceptance and inclusion of Buteyko's theory and his method of normalisation of breathing in primary management for asthma.

However, the trial and publication did get doctors and journalists talking about Buteyko and consequently members of the asthma public, worldwide, became aware. The Brisbane study was the impetus for interest and further trials in the United Kingdom and New Zealand. It has made Buteyko more accessible to people and has ultimately made a huge difference to the lives of thousands of people around the world.'

Dr. Simon Bowler, the doctor conducting the trial of Buteyko in Brisbane, had the trial article published in the Australian Medical Journal in December 1998. The results are summarised in the following table:

111

Measurement	Control Group	Buteyko Group
Breathing pattern at start	14.2 ± 4.9 L/min	14.0 ± 6.5 L/min
Breathing pattern at 3 months	13.3 ± 4.0 L/min	9.6 ± 3.1 L/min
End-tidal CO2 at start	32 ± 4 mm Hg	33 ± 5 mm Hg
End-tidal CO2 at 3 months	33 ± 3 mm Hg	35 ± 3 mm Hg
Preventer use at 3 months	Unchanged	49% av. reduction
Reliever use at 3 months	5% av. reduction	96% av. reduction
Quality of life at 3 months	0.4 improvement units	1.2 improvement units
Lung function tests at 3 months	Unchanged from start	Unchanged from start

Table 6.2. A summary of the Brisbane trial results of the Buteyko Method.

Some doctors negated the improvement in symptom and medication use because there was virtually no change in lung function tests. Tess Graham provides her reply to this and also gives another viewpoint to the results in the following report:

Self-Management of Asthma through Normalisation of Breathing - The Role of Breathing Therapy

The theory that hyperventilation and alveolar hypocapnia (low carbon dioxide pressure) is a major causal factor in asthma was shown to be correct in clinical trials funded by the Asthma Foundations of Australia, led by Professor Charles Mitchell and Dr. Simon Bowler.

It is well known that carbon dioxide is a bronchodilator and that deficiency can lead to bronchospasm. As early as 1932 Herxheimer treated patients with 5% carbon dioxide (Herxheimer 1952).

In a prospective double blind placebo controlled study the Buteyko Method was compared to conventional management of asthma. Forty asthmatics were split into two groups - one group was taught physiotherapy breathing exercises and the other the Buteyko Method.

- All subjects had asthma.
- All subjects showed hyperventilation.
- All subjects showed hypocapnia.
- All subjects were instructed to use bronchodilators on an "as needed" basis.
- The supervising doctor reduced steroid preventer medication on instruction.
- The average subject age was 47 years and each one had asthma duration for an average range of 23 years. This is relatively old and chronic with respect to most asthma studies.
- Buteyko subjects reduced their hyperventilation by an average of 31% in their minute volume at twelve weeks. There was no significant change in the control group (those practising physiotherapy exercises).
- There was a correlation between the relative reduction in need for bronchodilators and the proportionate reduction in minute volumes in Buteyko subjects; that is, the subject's need for bronchodilator medication was related to the volume of air they breathed. The more air an individual breathed, the more bronchodilator that person needed.
- In the initial twelve weeks of the study neither group had any significant change in the FEV_1 lung function. They maintained, on average, the previous personal best function. In the Buteyko group, this occurred along with an average 49% reduction in steroids and 90% reduction in their need for bronchodilators. The control group continued to require all their medication. The FEV_1 test relates to the number of years of asthma. Therefore, with subjects who have suffered asthma up to 60 years, dramatic improvements in lung function cannot be expected in just a 12-week period. The tendency for the FEV_1 test itself to provoke bronchospasm is related to the years of asthma.
- The Buteyko group significantly improved their quality of life compared to the control group. Buteyko subjects experienced a 71% reduction in symptoms. The control group had no significant change in asthma symptoms.
- Those who learned the Buteyko Method were able to maintain their reduction of bronchodilators by an average of 81% and their inhaled steroids by 28% in month eight of the study (winter time). At the same point, those on the conventional management programme had increased their use of bronchodilators by 28% and their inhaled steroids by 4%.

[Courtesy of Tess Graham]

References

Adams FV. The Asthma Sourcebook. Everything You Need to Know. Lowell House. Los Angeles. 1998. p48

Ameisen Paul J. Every Breath You Take. Tandem Press. 1997. p111

Anderson Price S, McCarty Wilson L. Pathophysiology. Clinical concepts of Disease Processes. Fourth Edition. Mosby. St. Louis. 1992. pp117, 118, 122, 124

Asher MI, Greening AP. Drug Use in Respiratory Disease. Williams & Wilkins. Sydney. 1987. pp241, 244

Bowler SD et al. Buteyko breathing techniques in asthma: a blinded randomised controlled trial. MJA 1998. 169. pp575-578

Brisco P. Youngsen. R. Asthma: Questions You Have – Answers You Need. Thorsons. 1997. p73

Castle W, Fuller R, Hall J, Palmer J. Serevent nationwide surveillance study: comparison of Salmeterol with Salbutamol in asthmatic patients who require regular bronchodilator treatment. BMJ. 1993. 306. pp1034-1037

Cochrane GM. Drug Use in Respiratory Disease. Williams & Wilkins. Sydney. 1987. p100

Crane J, Burgess C, Pearce N, Beasley R. The beta-agonist controversy: a perspective. European. Respiratory. Reve. 1993. 3. pp475-482

Crane J, Pearce N, Flatt A et al. Prescribed Fenoterol and death from asthma in New Zealand, 1981-1983: a case control study. Lancet 1989. 1. pp917-922

Deal FC, McFadden ER, Ingram RH, Strauss RH, Jaegger JJ. Role of respiratory heat exchange in production of exercise induced asthma. J Applied Phys. 1979. 46. pp467-475

Downes S, article from Airways, summarised in: The beta agonist debate - new insights. The Asthma Welfarer 1995. 29. pp1-3

Fried R. The Psychology and Physiology of Breathing. Plenum Press. New York 1993. p289

Gardner WN. The Pathophysiology of Hyperventilation Disorders. Chest 1996. 109. pp516-534

Grampian Asthma Study of Integrated Care. Integrated Care for Asthmatics. BMJ. 1994. 308. pp559-564

Grippi M. Pulmonary Pathophysiology. J.B. Lippincott Company. Philadelphia. 1995. p249

Graham T. Self Management of Asthma through Normalisation of Breathing – The Role of Breathing Therapy. 1996.

Groen JJ. The psychosomatic theory of bronchial asthma. Psychother Psychosom 1979. 31. pp38-48

Haas F, Sperber Haas S. The Essential Asthma Book. Ivy Books. New York. 1994. pp268, 270

Herxheimer H.G. The Management of Bronchial Asthma. London. 1952.

Hibbert GA, Pilsbury DJ. Demonstration and treatment of hyperventilation causing asthma. British J Psych. 1988. 53. pp687-689

Holgate ST. Asthma and Allergy – disorders of civilization? QJM. 1998. 91. pp171-184

Holt S. Asthma in New Zealand: myths and realities. NZ Medical J. Feb 11, 2000. pp39–41

Hough A. Physiotherapy in Respiratory Care. Stanley Thornes Ltd. London. 1997. pp60, 61, 67, 100

Inman WHN, Adelstein AM. Rise and fall of asthma mortality in England and Wales in relation to use of pressurized aerosols. Lancet. 1969. 2. pp279-283

Jackson RT, Beaglehole R. Rea HH, Sutherland DC. Mortality from asthma: a new epidemic in New Zealand. BMJ. 1982. 285. pp771-774

Juniper EF, Kline PA, Vanzieleghem MA, Ramsdale EH, O'Byrne PM, Hargreave FE. Effect of Long-term treatment with an inhaled corticosteroids (budesonide) on airway hyper-responsiveness and clinical asthma in non-steroid dependant asthmatics. Am Rev Respir Dis 1990. 142. pp832-836

Kontos HA, Richardson DW, Raper AJ, Zubair-Ul-Hassan, Patterson JL. Mechanisms of action of hypocapnic alkalosis on limb blood vessels in man and dog. Am J Physiology. Dec 1972. 223. pp1296-1307

Lim TK, Ang SM, Rossing TH et al. The effects of deep inhalation on maximal expiratory flow during spontaneous asthmatic episodes. Am Rev Respir Dis. 1989. 140. pp340-343

Lum L.C. Behavioural and Psychological Approaches to Breathing Disorders. Ed. B.H. Timmons & R Ley. New York. Plenum. 1994. pp115-116

Lumb AB. Nunn's Applied Respiratory Physiology. Reed. London. 2000. pp23, 26, 530

McFadden ER, Lyons HA. Arterial blood gas tension in asthma. N. Eng. J Medicine. 1968. 278. pp1027-1032

McIvor RA, Pizzichini E. Turner MO, Hussack P, Hargreaves FE, Sears MR. Potential masking effects of salmeterol on airway inflammation in asthma. Am J Respiratory & Critical Care Medicine. 1998 Sep. 158(3). pp924-930

Milne C. Treating athletes with Asthma. New Ethicals 1996 Jan. 33. 1. pp9-17.

National Asthma Education Program. Expert Panel Report. Guidelines for the Diagnostics and Management of Asthma. Bethesda, Md: National Institute of Health, 1991. US Dept. of Health and Human Services Publication. PHS. 91-3042

Neville E, Gribbins H, Harrison BDW. Acute severe asthma. Respir Medicine. 1991. 85. pp463-474

Schuster A, Kizlik R, Reinhardt D. Influence of short and long term inhalation of Salbutamol on lung function and beta2-adrenoreceptors of mononuclear blood vessels in asthmatic children. European. J Pediatrics. 1991. 150. pp209-213

Sears MR, Taylor DR. Regular Beta-agonist therapy – The quality of the evidence. European Respiratory J. 1992. 5. pp896-897

Sears MR, Taylor DR, Print CG, et al. Regular inhaled beta-agonist treatment in asthma. Lancet. 1990. 336. pp1391-1396

Smyth ET, Pavord ID, Wong CS, Wisniewski AF, Williams J, Tattersfield AE. Interaction and dose equivalence of salbutamol and salmeterol in patients with asthma. BMJ. 1993. 306. pp543-545

Speizer FE, Doll R, Heaf P, Strang LB. Investigation into use of drugs preceding deaths from asthma. BMJ. 1968.1. pp339-343

Thompson Bernice. Better Breathing. Simple Exercises for the Relief of Asthma, Bronchitis and Emphysema. Pegasus. Christchurch. 1967. p14

van den Elshout F, van Herwaarden J, Folgering H. Effects of hypercapnia and hypocapnia on respiratory resistance in normal and asthmatic subjects. Thorax. 1991. 46. pp28-32

It is believed by Buteyko proponents that everyone with asthma hyperventilates, but not everyone who hyperventilates has asthma.

Like the food that we eat, breathing affects every cell in the entire body and just as overeating does not provide good health, neither does over-breathing. As the Disease of Deep Breathing is investigated it is noted that a number of health problems arise in different individuals, which is possibly due to both nature and nurture. The next section of this book discusses other conditions that are related to the Disease of Deep Breathing and the Carbon Dioxide Syndrome.

Chapter 7

Insomnia, Snoring and Sleep Apnoea

Sleeping soundly is so important to those who do not enjoy this basic need, that they will go to extraordinary lengths to achieve it.

People who hyperventilate will be familiar with some of the following indicators of poor sleep:

- Repeatedly waking during the night
- Waking up tired instead of refreshed
- Vivid dreams and nightmares
- Night sweats
- Having extra mucus in the morning
- Talking or walking during sleep.

People who sleep with those who hyperventilate will also be aware of other factors such as snoring, sleep apnoea, having the blankets tossed about the bed all night. It seems that when people sleep badly, everyone is affected.

Hot chocolate contains caffeine but is considered perfectly acceptable to induce sleep, yet when a person has trouble sleeping caffeine is something that is often blamed, along with too much light or noise. However, when someone is really tired, they fall asleep anywhere, even while reading, watching television, during a meeting or on a train in rush hour.

Does This Sound Familiar?

You lie down to sleep, close your eyes and drift off, sleeping soundly for several hours. When it is time to get up, you jump out of bed, feeling great, ready for the new day.

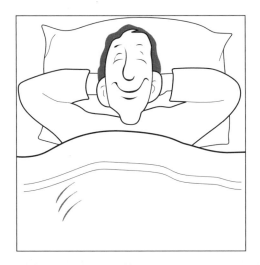

Or Is This More Like It?

You are so exhausted that you fall asleep immediately, only to wake three or four hours later with a dry mouth and needing to go to the bathroom. If you have asthma, then you probably also need a puff of your reliever. Now you are restless, not really asleep, yet not awake either and deep sleep only comes again when it is close to the time to get up. Consequently in the morning you feel tired and perhaps even worse than when you went to bed.

This is the common sleep pattern for people who hyperventilate. If this isn't bad enough, the person also wakes up with a dry, foul tasting mouth, bad breath and a blocked nose. 'I NEVER get enough sleep!' is the common complaint, while they cough or blow their nose through half a box of tissues.

Sound Sleep

As a person relaxes and prepares for sleep, the breathing pattern lessens slightly, creating a small rise in carbon dioxide. This might be resisted at first with repeated yawning, but after a time the respiratory centre adjusts to the lower pH and the nervous system relaxes, encouraging sleep (Jennet 1994). To remain asleep, this small rise in the pressure of carbon dioxide needs to be maintained.

When babies are asleep, their breathing is so gentle that it is hard to see any movement and this is the way that everyone should breathe when sleeping. To meet the demands of metabolism during sleep, it is only necessary to breathe through one nostril, and this is normally achieved by lying on one side. The nostril that is closest to the pillow fills with fluid while the other is breathed through. When the working nostril gets tired, it causes the person to roll over and the reverse happens (Cole 1984). This cycle is repeated several times a night and ensures a sound sleep because backache, cramp, numbness and circulatory problems (Davies 1989) can occur if the person stays in one position for too long.

Poor Sleep Patterns

Being able to breathe through your nose therefore is vital for a sound sleep because with a chronically blocked nose it is impossible to maintain this cycle (Barelli 1994). The fastest way to block up the nose is to breathe too much air, especially through the mouth, which is why lying on the back tends to encourage poor sleep patterns. In this position the jaw is likely to relax so much that the mouth falls open and facilitates the loss of carbon dioxide, as well as heat and water from the lungs, throat and mouth. The lungs are large organs – if they could be spread out they would be approximately the same size as a tennis court – and they are filled with tiny blood vessels, which make them heavy. When lying on the back, breathing muscles have to work harder to move air in and out of the lungs (Hough 1997) and the effort of this requires additional oxygen as well as ridding the body of extra carbon dioxide. This removes the sleepy, relaxed feeling that a higher pressure of carbon dioxide provides and either wakes the person up or prevents them from getting to sleep in the first place.

Simultaneously, smooth muscle spasms, and this may cause reactions such as chest tightness or an urge to empty the bladder. In an effort to balance the pH of the blood, kidneys excrete bicarbonate ions, which also make more frequent urination. Other electrolytes such as magnesium, calcium, potassium and sodium also play a part in balancing the pH and as their normal levels alter, a variety of changes take place. None of these factors are conducive to sound sleep.

It would seem that sleeping flat on the back is a relatively new experience as it was only a few centuries ago that many people slept virtually sitting up to cope with the smoky atmosphere of homes that had inadequate chimneys. Since it is more difficult to breathe while lying on the back than lying on one side, it does not seem a particularly good practice to encourage.

Insomnia

Constantly feeling tired and battling with sleep each night not only encourages health risks but it can also make the rest of your life harder to cope with. So people who lack sleep often crave it, spending eight to ten hours in bed at a stretch whenever they can. There is no proof that this is healthy and in fact a study conducted in the United States on over one million adults by Dr. Daniel Kripke and his peers (2002). It was revealed that people who sleep for eight hours or more die at a younger age than those who sleep a little less. The professor of psychiatry at the University of California in San Diego was reported in the Evening Post Wellington (2002) as saying, "Individuals who now average six and a half hours of sleep a night can be reassured that this is a safe amount of sleep. From a health standpoint there is no reason to sleep longer." This is one very good reason to stop building frustration next time you are wide-awake and wishing that you were asleep.

Having poor sleep patterns not only makes a person tired but also they are often accompanied by the more harmful conditions of snoring or sleep apnoea.

Snoring

Since breathing through the mouth is unnatural when sleeping, then breathing through the mouth so vigorously that you make a noise is even more so. Anyone can snore if they have a cold, nasal polyps, a nasal infection or enlarged adenoids, but it seems to be primarily linked to obesity, aging and alcohol. Men snore even more than women (Guilleminault 1994, Lumb 2000).

The person doing the snoring usually feels that they have slept quite soundly but it is the effects of snoring that are not healthy. As well as making the person feel rather tired and perhaps guilty for waking other people, snoring can also cause health problems such as hypertension, heart and chest disease, rheumatism, diabetes and depression (Lumb 2000).

Sleep Apnoea

Snoring night after night often develops into the more serious sleep apnoea. Sleep apnoea means that while sleeping, the person has periods of breathing quite vigorously and periods of not breathing at all (apnoea). There are two major and overlapping causes of sleep apnoea – obstruction of the airways and a reduction in the drive to breathe.

During sleep there are two types of sleep patterns – Rapid Eye Movement (REM), which is when dreaming occurs and non-REM (NREM), the deep, dreamless period of sleep. During NREM, which is approximately 80% of sleep time (Tortora 1984), breathing is critically dependent on carbon dioxide pressure. As soon as the pressure drops, the breathing stops until it builds up sufficiently to initiate the next breath (Skatrud 1983, Xie 1995).

Like snoring, sleep apnoea tends to get worse as the person gets older, fatter or after drinking alcohol. Getting worse means more episodes of apnoea, which in some cases are short but reach up to 160 times per hour, while others are less frequent but can be as much as 90 seconds long. To stop breathing 300 – 400 times in a night for at least ten seconds is common in people with sleep apnoea (Davies 1993, Lumb 2000). Even though the sufferer does not consciously wake up each time, sleep is not sound either. The primary danger from sleep apnoea is that both oxygen and carbon dioxide pressures are abnormally low. It has been linked to the same health problems as snoring and also a diminished ability to think clearly or remember things, headaches, impotence, daytime fatigue which can sometimes be so severe that the person will fall asleep while driving a car, emotional and often irrational behaviour such as jealousy, suspicion, hostility and paranoia (Davies 1993, Lumb 2000).

Partners of people with sleep apnoea typically also sleep badly because if the snoring does not wake them then the silence does. A thirty second pause in breathing seems a very long time, and the partner may worry that the person is never going to start breathing again.

Sleep Better

To achieve a good night's sleep, you need to breathe quietly through your nose, preferably while lying on one side. Breathing is never more automatic than during sleep and the way to correct a hyperventilation-related problem is to normalise the respiratory centre's setting of carbon dioxide. Breathing then becomes acceptable for any activity, including sleep. Some of the things that people try in an effort to sleep more soundly include:

- Wearing nasal strips to facilitate nasal-breathing.
- Wearing a small backpack or sewing a tennis ball into the back of their pyjama coat to encourage sleeping on one side.
- Getting someone to watch you sleep, rolling you over and closing your mouth when necessary.
- Wearing a chin-strap like Hercule Poirot, a mouth-guard, or taping their mouth closed.
- Having surgery to trim the soft palate or move the jaw forward.
- Using a Continuous Positive Air Pressure (CPAP) machine to send a continuous pressure of air through the airways to prevent them from collapsing.

A person who is willing to have surgery in order to sleep well demonstrates how important getting sound sleep is. Part of the Buteyko way to help this problem is to encourage sleeping on one side and to tape the mouth closed. This does not mean putting masking tape "hostage-style" across the mouth but placing a narrow piece of surgical paper tape, nose to chin direction across the lips. The aim is to encourage breathing through the nose rather than to prevent mouth breathing. When a small piece of tape placed loosely across the centre of the mouth is used alongside the thought, 'I want to breathe through my nose', it helps to achieve this aim because it prevents the jaw from relaxing completely when rolling onto the back.

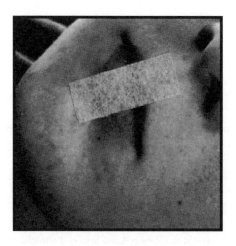

Figure 7:1. Loosely taping your mouth helps to encourage breathing through the nose during sleep.

If your nose is stuffy, then get it clear before putting the tape on by using the Nose Clearing exercise in chapter four or another successful method. Once the mouth is taped and you are comfortable breathing through your nose, then decide which nostril is the most blocked and roll onto that side so that the blocked nostril is closest to the pillow. Continue to breathe easily and without any effort from your breathing muscles.

WARNING: Taping the mouth closed, even in a non-threatening way as suggested here, can be frightening for some people. Because of this, even loosely taping the mouth should NOT be attempted with:

- Babies or children under the age of four.
- People who suffer from claustrophobia.
- Anyone with a blocked nose.

'Since I've taped my 5-year-old's mouth at night, he sleeps better, has no asthma symptoms and is eating really well. He asks for it each night because he knows it works!' Patricia

References

Barelli P. Behavioural and Psychological Approaches to Breathing Disorders. Ed. B.H. Timmons & R Ley. Plenum. New York. 1994. p51

Cole P, Haight J.S Posture and nasal patency. American Review of Respiratory Diseases, 1984. 129. pp351 – 354

Davies AM, Koenig JS, Thach BT Characteristics of upper airway chemoreflex prolonged apnoea in human infants. Am Rev of Respiratory Dis. 1989. 139. pp668-673

Davies RJO, Stradling JR. Acute effects of obstructive sleep apnoea. British J Anasth. 1993. 71. pp725-729

Guilleminault C, Bliwise DL. Behavioural and Psychological Approaches to Breathing Disorders. Ed. B.H. Timmons & R Ley. New York. Plenum. 1994. p61

Hough A. Physiotherapy in Respiratory Care. Stanley Thornes Ltd. London . 1997. p7

Jennet S. Behavioural and Psychological Approaches to Breathing Disorders. Ed. B.H. Timmons & R Ley. New York. Plenum. 1994. p77

Kripke DF, Garfinkel L, Wingard DL, Klauber MR, Marier MR. Mortality Associated With Sleep Duration and Insomnia. Arch General Psychiatry. 2002. 59. pp131-136

Lumb AB. Nunn's Applied Respiratory Physiology. Reed. London. 2000. pp347, 348

'Sleep Late, die early, study shows'. Wake-up Call. Evening Post Wellington, New

Zealand. 15/02/02

Skatrud JB, Demsey JA. Interaction of sleep state and chemical stimuli in sustaining rhythmic ventilation. J Applied Physiology. 1983. 55. pp813-822

Tortora GJ, Anagnostakos NP. Principles of Anatomy and Physiology, Harper & Row, New York. 1984. p358

Xie A, Rutherford R, Rankin F, Wong B, Bradley TD. Hypocapnia and Increased Ventilatory Responsiveness in Patients with Idiopathic Central Sleep Apnea. Am J. Respir. Critical. Care Medicine 1995. 152. pp1950-1955

Chapter 8

Allergies and Nasal Problems

Rhinitis and sinus problems are very like asthma, except that the problem is in the nose instead of in the chest.

When exposed to dangers such as bacteria and chemicals, the nasal passages automatically swell and produce more mucus, which is useful to keep out poisonous gases but annoying when patting a cat. Sometimes the immune system malfunctions and recognises harmless agents, like cat dander or pollen, as potential dangers. It is the body's overreaction to the cat dander that is causes the problem, rather than the actual cat dander. Histamines spring into action, causing swelling, itching, smooth muscle contraction, leaky blood vessels and a rise in mucus production.

Allergy sufferers are familiar with the 'Allergic Salute', when the end of the nose is pushed upwards to open the nasal passages and to alleviate the itchiness, and also 'Allergic Shiners', those dark shadows under the eyes that make you look as if you haven't slept in a week. Glassy, red eyes usually complete the picture of the allergic rhinitis sufferer.

As well as causing irritation and a localised immune response, inhaling allergens is a stress that affects the whole body. While it is not life threatening to walk around with several tissues in your pocket, the constant sneezing, running nose, tickle in the throat and cough are extremely tiresome. This on its own is likely to increase breathing and raise blood pressure. Added to this is the fact that allergens are often in the air for weeks at a time. For example, a person may be particularly sensitive to pine tree pollen that floats around for at least two months in springtime. Because the person is under stress and consequently breathing more than usual for this entire time, extra allergens are inhaled and more carbon dioxide is lost, turning the situation into a vicious circle.

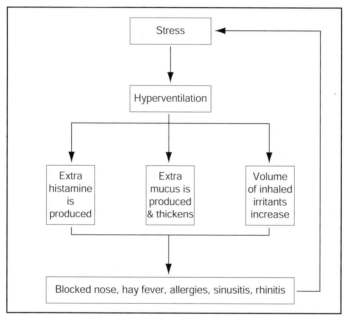

Figure 8:1. The cycle of hyperventilation and nasal problems often seem never ending.

It is a basic Buteyko belief that the nose is the first line of defence against hyperventilation, and also against invasion by foreign particles since it is both the start of the respiratory tract and the body part especially designed for breathing. When breathing more air than is required, the nose blocks to slow the loss of carbon dioxide. Not being aware of this, the person unfortunately breathes harder or starts using his or her mouth.

If the problem of hypocapnia is not resolved, the nose often remains blocked, escalating the situation because low carbon dioxide stimulates histamine production. The narrowed nasal passages restrict normal flow of mucus and the extra breathing dries mucus, making it harder to shift and less effective against infection. Taking anti-allergy tablets, nasal dilators or antibiotics seem to help at first but their effectiveness diminishes and some medications have a rebound effect, making symptoms worse. Combine these issues with the fact that chronic hyperventilation can suppress the immune system (Timmons 1994) and the result can be a painful sinus infection or at best, a chronically blocked nose.

Stop Sneezing

Having rhinitis or hay fever is rather like having asthma; you have narrowed airways and copious mucus, except that the problem is in your nose instead of in your lungs. Bearing this in mind, you might find that following the rules regarding asthma medications could be useful. Do not overdose with relievers, and take nasal steroid medications to dampen down the symptoms if the use of relievers is getting out of hand.

Eliminating the irritants that initiate your reaction seems an obvious answer, but if it is not possible to eliminate them then perhaps wearing a mask when around them may be helpful. However, triggers are not always obvious, so keeping a diary of your diet, activities and weather patterns could be useful in pinpointing what promotes your problem.

To make positive changes without using drugs by normalising your breathing pattern would be another good place to start because:

- When a normal amount of carbon dioxide is retained, there is no need for the protective mechanism of narrowing nasal passages to reduce the loss.
- Fewer irritants are inhaled.
- Excessive histamine production is reduced, which results in less inflammation and mucus production.
- By breathing less the protective mucus does not dry out, which means that mucus glands do not pump out excessive mucus to keep the nose moist and the mucus is not as thick.
- Mucus is able to move freely because nasal passages are open.
- The immune system works more efficiently.

'I used Ventolin at least five times a day before I attended a Buteyko course two years ago. My hay fever and allergies made life hell. I haven't used Ventolin on a regular basis since about one month after the course. My energy, motivation and self-esteem have improved. Buteyko enabled me to exercise and so I lost weight and became fitter and healthier. I have 98% less hay fever and my skin is healthier - I have less eczema.' Madeline

References
Timmons BH. Behavioural and Psychological Approaches to Breathing Disorders. Ed. B.H. Timmons & R Ley. Plenum. New York. 1994. p263

Chapter 9

Eczema and Itchy Skin

Allergies do not only affect the airways, but also sometimes react with the skin causing eczema, itchy skin or rashes. While having an itch that will not go away is not life-threatening, it is extremely debilitating.

The skin is the largest organ and since it is on the outside of the body it comes into contact with many stressors, such as pollutants, germs and too much sun. Factors from outside the body are not the only things to irritate the skin. Some body wastes are removed through perspiration (Tortora 1984) and it is common in people with eczema to feel that they react to their own sweat.

It is also easy for the skin to receive insufficient blood and nutrients because a primary function of the skin is to assist in maintaining a constant body temperature of 37° Celsius. When the air is cool, such as when working in an air-conditioned building, blood flow to the skin reduces to prevent loss of heat. When faced with danger, blood flow to the skin also reduces to minimise potential bleeding, which in the short-term is useful. However, hidden hyperventilation also results in less blood flow and nourishment to the skin and unlike the fight or flight response, it can be maintained for years. Long-term, this may lead to a chronically pale complexion, cold extremities, malfunction of tissue cells and premature aging.

Hidden hyperventilation and the resulting hypocapnia triggers histamine production (Kontos 1972). Swelling occurs and tiny blood vessels become leaky, which may show as redness or other discoloration. Histamine can also cause itching, inflammation and a rash. Sometimes the urge to scratch is so great that the person scratches until they bleed and then scratches a little more, knowing all the time that they are harming their skin, yet unable to stop. The sense of frustration and self-defeat only contributes to the already stressful situation.

Approximately one and a half litres of water is supplied each day by the nose to moisten inhaled air (Fried 1987) and water vapour is exhaled, so if a person breathes faster than normal without drinking extra water to compensate, this could dehydrate the body and lead to dry, flaky skin.

Hormones are substances created by the body to regulate normal bodily functions, and like every other part of the body, the glands that make these hormones are affected by breathing. A classic example is the increased production of adrenaline by the adrenal glands when the fight or flight response is initiated. However, all hormones are affected by breathing, including those that control the growth of hair and skin, the repair of skin and so on. If the glands that produce these hormones do not receive sufficient oxygen or the pH of their intracellular fluid is not ideal, then their function will be less than perfect. This can result in a number of problems, which include poor healing, discoloration, coarseness of skin and hair loss.

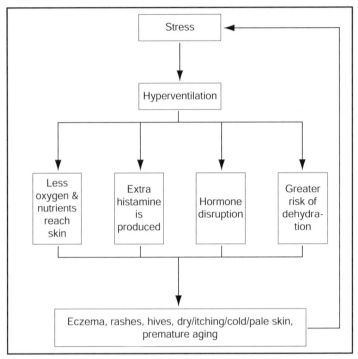

Figure 9:1. The connection between stress and irritated skin.

Get Rid of the Itch

All of the above make the skin extra sensitive and things that were not irritating before may become so now. To change this you can try a number of things:

- Avoid putting very hot water, perfumes or any kind of irritant on your skin as these only stress the already sensitive skin.
- Drink plenty of water to avoid dehydration.
- Topical steroid creams or oral steroids may be required from time to time to short circuit the immune system's overreaction to irritants, but be careful how and where

you use them as they may also cause permanent damage to the skin.

- Keep a diary of foods that you eat and creams that you apply to the skin to see if there is a connection to the irritation.

- Scratching only causes more of a problem by irritating the skin. You can demonstrate this by dragging a fingernail firmly along your inner arm and watching for the red mark that appears within a minute. Rub gently when the itch is annoying, but try not to scratch.

- Resume normal breathing patterns, which should improve blood flow, moisture to the skin and a drop in histamine levels. This will mean an improvement in skin colouring, less itching and warmer extremities. The change in skin colouring and texture is often dramatic.

'My nose was permanently blocked and my skin terribly itchy - my fingers cracked and bled so that I had to wear band aids by day and plastic gloves over ointment by night. By day four, my condition had improved as if I had taken a short sharp course of Prednisone (without the health risk). I could smell the grass and my fingers and cheeks felt warm and I had stopped scratching.'
Dennis

References

Fried R. The Hyperventilation Syndrome Research and Clinical Treatment. The John Hopkins University Press. 1987. p11

Kontos HA, Richardson DW, Raper AJ, Zubair-Ul-Hassan, Patterson JL. Mechanisms of action of hypocapnic alkalosis on limb blood vessels in man and dog. Am J Physiology. Dec 1972. 223. pp1296-1307

Tortora GJ, Anagnostakos NP. Principles of Anatomy and Physiology, Harper & Row, New York. 1984. p113

Chapter 10

Lacking Energy

Taking part in regular physical exercise is a vital component to good health. However, for many people this seems an impossible task because they either lack the strength or it creates so many negative symptoms that it does not appear to be worth the effort.

When there is insufficient breath to run, it is hard to be team captain and sometimes even too hard to participate. Even though very few people will be Olympians, participation in regular exercise is one of the keys to good health because exercise increases the heart and breathing rates, causes perspiration and at the same time strengthens muscles and bones, while releasing tension and toxins. It should be enjoyable and invigorating so that afterwards you feel glad that you participated. Creating exhaustion or breathing difficulties by doing exercise that is too vigorous or too prolonged is not a sensible approach.

Buteyko Practitioners strongly promote physical exercise because it is one way of increasing carbon dioxide levels as well as creating a healthier lifestyle and a sense of wellbeing. However, exercise should be at the level where breathing is still relatively comfortably, or there is a risk of removing more carbon dioxide than is being produced.

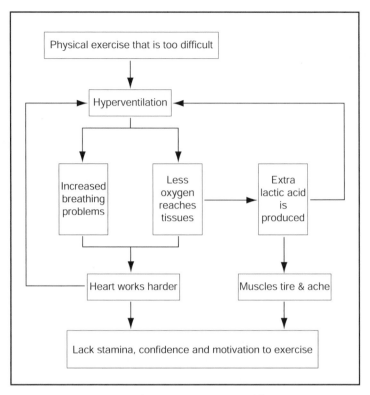

Figure 10:1. Doing too much exercise creates problems.

The Vicious Circle of Exercise

While doing too much exercise can cause problems, so does doing little or no physical exercise. Until the past few decades, people did not go to the gym to get fit because there was no need to. Most people exercised for several hours every day by walking, biking, horse-riding, digging, washing clothes or sweeping floors. These activities require muscle movement and were a normal part of everyday life. Over time, lifestyles in developed countries have become increasingly sedentary with most people no longer living and working in small villages where everything is within walking distance, and today most families own a car.

Doing little or no exercise diminishes general fitness and encourages weight gain, which places a greater strain on the heart and lungs when exercise is attempted, tiring the body more quickly. Exercise consequently seems less possible or desirable, and so the walking shoes get pulled out even less often, while health problems mount up.

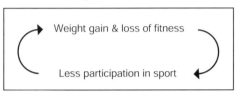

Weight gain & loss of fitness

Less participation in sport

Figure 10:2. Not doing enough exercise also creates problems.

In despair of this vicious cycle, many people stop exercising totally and find that the only time they walk is from the car into the shopping centre. Carparks closest to the entrance are always the ones filled first at malls and even at gyms or swimming pools where the sole purpose of going is to get fit. The average adult of today in any western country weighs far more than the average adult of eighty years ago, and one of the most likely reasons for this is the lack of exercise that accompanies today's lifestyle.

Break Out of the Circle

'When Benjamin completed the Buteyko course many people commented on the tremendous improvement in his rugby. We had thought that he was a bit frightened of the action and hung back but after learning Buteyko there was no holding him. We realise now that he had no breath and energy to keep up.' Alison (Mother)

When muscles move they produce lots of carbon dioxide, which helps to maintain the normal volume that is required to stay healthy. However, a sharp build-up of carbon dioxide stimulates the breathing pattern, making it possible to breathe more than one hundred litres of air each minute during exercise (Salazah 1991). Therefore, it is just as important to breathe only as much as metabolism requires at this time as it is while doing any other activity.

When commencing an exercise programme for the first time in many years it is advisable to visit your doctor for a general checkup to ensure that your whole body is working the way it should. Take the time to rest when you are tired and go easy on yourself. When you are able to cope with gentle exercise, then go a little faster, further, or add a hill to your regime, but never make it so difficult that you need to open your mouth to breathe. People who already exercise regularly would also be wise to slow their pace for a week or two so that they are able to breathe easily through their nose. Learning to control your breathing reduces or eliminates symptoms of breathlessness (Hibbert 1988) and within a short time you will find exercise more enjoyable.

It is noticeable that in the animal kingdom virtually no animal voluntarily runs until it needs to breathe through its mouth. Instead, it slows down or stops as it tires, continuing to breathe through its nose or perhaps panting for a short time to cool down before returning to nose-breathing almost immediately. People on the other hand often go as fast as they can, even if it means mouth-breathing to do so, instead of letting their breathing be the guide as to how fast they can move. When you already have asthma symptoms or sensitive, irritated airways, it makes even less sense to breathe through your mouth. Nose-breathing the whole time and letting a sense of ease with your breathing decide the pace are the first steps towards making an improvement in your sporting ability.

Asthmatics who take reliever medication so that they can exercise are acting like a person who twists his ankle, takes painkillers, and straps the ankle to keep running. When treating an inflamed ankle you normally rest, take anti-inflammatory medication and as you heal, start a gentle exercise programme to rebuild fitness. Since the underlying cause of asthma is currently believed to be inflammation in the airways, it is unlikely that it should be treated any differently. Taking reliever so that you can exercise is more likely to aggravate the situation.

Heat and moisture are lost during exercise, not only from the airways but from the whole body. Dehydration is not conducive to good health because approximately 60% of body weight or 40 litres of water is required for the healthy function of the adult body (Sukkar 1993). For example, water is required to lubricate the joints and if the alveoli are not moist then oxygen cannot dissolve and pass into the bloodstream (Tortora 1984). It is therefore very important to keep the fluid intake up, both during and after exercise.

When insufficient oxygen is released to tissue cells, lactic acid builds up and muscles tire quickly. This is a self-protective mechanism that causes the person to slow down or stop so that muscle tissue is not damaged. Those who believe in the old adage of 'No pain, no gain', and try to push through the pain barrier in an effort to get fit quickly invariably get injuries. Paying attention to your body and working within your capabilities is a much safer way of improving fitness.

'Buteyko has given me new hope for fitness into old age, with much more controlled breathing. I weigh less and have much more stable energy levels. I no longer fear moderate exercise and my muscles are much more relaxed.' Basil

References

Hibbert GA, Pilsbury DJ. Demonstration and treatment of hyperventilation causing asthma. British J Psych. 1988. 153. pp687-689

Salazah J. Exercise physiology, in Pulmonary Therapy and Rehabilitation. Eds. Haas F, Axen K. Williams and Wilkins. Baltimore. 1991. pp58, 63

Sukkar MY, El-Munshid HA & Ardawi. Concise Human Physiology. Blackwell Scientific Publications. Oxford. 1993. p6

Tortora GJ, Anagnostakos NP. Principles of Anatomy and Physiology, Harper & Row, New York. 1984. p38

Chapter 11

M.E. or C.F.S.

While not being able to take part fully in sport is frustrating, it is infinitely preferable to having Chronic Fatigue Syndrome (C.F.S.) or Myalgic Encephalomyelitis (M.E.) which leaves the person feeling tired almost all of the time and suffering from a wide range of symptoms. Physical activities that were previously done easily now cause extreme fatigue that may take hours or even days to recover from. Mental tasks are also taxing.

'My M.E./C.F.S. started with what seemed like five separate flu infections in six weeks. My immune system appeared to be destroyed because I picked up infections very easily over the next few years. I felt exhausted most of the time. I slept fifteen hours a day, and just managed to look after myself in the remaining seven. My brain seemed to have shut down, my short-term memory disappeared, and I couldn't read newspapers, paperwork or books, because I just couldn't understand them. The only thing I could follow was daytime TV. When I walked it felt like I was wading through treacle, and I often needed a rest walking up one flight of stairs. I felt like an old woman but I was only thirty.' Sally

In the past, people with this syndrome were often thought of as malingerers or hypochondriacs. Diagnosis was difficult because there were no analysis criteria for doctors to rely on, but in 1994 a group of Chronic Fatigue Syndrome researchers (Fukuda et al) set down the following as a diagnostic aid:

1. The person must have had severe and chronic fatigue for at least six months and no other medical conditions found. Conditions which have similar symptoms include: sleep

apnoea, hypothyroidism, severe depression, schizophrenia, eating disorders, cancer, autoimmune disease, chronic low grade infection and obesity. These must be ruled out.

2. At least four of the following eight symptoms must have appeared and be present at the same time during this period:

- Impairment of short-term memory or concentration.
- Waking up tired even after a good sleep.
- Tender lymph glands.
- Muscle pain.
- Pain without swelling or redness in more than one joint.
- Headaches of a new type, pattern or severity.
- Sore throat.
- Not feeling well for more than twenty-four hours after doing physical exercise or exertion.

Who Gets M.E./C.F.S?

M.E./C.F.S. mostly affects young adults aged between twenty and forty years of age, but it can also be found in children and teenagers. The incidence is not related to any particular social group but women suffer more frequently from this condition than men (Lloyd 1990).

Why M.E./C.F.S. Occurs

A major stress such as illness, toxic overload or viral infection usually occurs before M.E./C.F.S. starts, but there is no one thing common to all sufferers and many people experience similar events without developing the syndrome, which leaves the exact source a mystery to medical science.

Hans Selye, the doctor who discovered that stress causes physical reactions, may be able to explain why it happens. In his book "Stress of Life" (1984) he proposed that people are born with a kind of 'adaptation energy' or an energy bank:

> 'It is as though, at birth, each individual inherited a certain amount of adaptation energy, the magnitude of which is determined by his genetic background, his parents... In any case, there is just so much of it, and he must budget accordingly.'

It is possible to make both deposits and withdrawals to this energy bank. Every time a person gets under stress, they make a withdrawal and when they rest, have fun, eat wholesome food or do other good things for their health and well being, they make a deposit. The deposits are never quite as much as the withdrawals and so when the end of the total deposit is finally reached, the person dies. It is possible that those with M.E./ C.F.S. have less adaptation energy than the norm, but not that they are more likely to die sooner than others, just that their need to rest arrives earlier.

As mentioned in Chapter One, Selye provided medicine with the accepted theory that the reaction to any stressful situation has three parts:

1.   The alarm reaction
2.   The stage of resistance
3.   The stage of exhaustion

These stages are repeated over and over in a lifetime and the stage of exhaustion does not necessarily mean death, just that it is time to stop doing the activity. For example, when going for a run the body has to work hard at first while the leg and arm muscles warm up and the heart gets pumping (alarm reaction).

Once the body has adapted, and especially if the person is fit, it is easy to run for quite some time (resistance stage), but even the fittest person will get tired arms and legs eventually and need to take a break (stage of exhaustion). After taking a rest however, the person can run again.

This can be applied to life in general where numerous stressors are thrust upon people – all creating a little 'wear and tear' – and insufficient deposits are made to counteract them. Because of the constant stress, breathing is always slightly increased, which is not life threatening but causes a number of things to occur that explain the symptoms of this condition. For example, blood flow to the brain drops, lowering oxygen and glucose delivery, creating cognitive problems (Ley 1994) where even simple mathematical problems seem difficult, or things are easily forgotten. Headaches could also be caused by lack of oxygen or perhaps hyperventilation-related muscle tension.

Because the fight or flight response is frequently being switched on to deal with situations that it is not designed to cope with, the adrenal glands work extra hard to continue to produce adrenaline in order to respond to these perceived dangers. This gland must also suffer from the General Adaptation Syndrome: at first responding quickly and effectively, but after several years of overuse, with less speed. Perhaps it gets to the point where it only responds after a lengthy period, and even then ineffectively, like starting a car which has a half-flat battery.

A small drop in carbon dioxide raises the pH inside nerve cells, stimulating their action. At first the person moves faster and is more aware of noises and lights, but if hyperventilation continues and the carbon dioxide pressure drops further, nerve cell activity slows as lactic acid production increases (Lum 1994).

If carbon dioxide continues dropping with still more lactic acid being produced, then the nerve cell activity can virtually stop altogether and in extreme cases the person becomes comatose (Lum 1978). While not in this severe condition, tissues receiving less oxygen and producing extra lactic acid cause the person to have tired and sore muscles as well as a great urge to slow down, rest and allow the body to recover. Today's busy lifestyle often dictates a nonstop treadmill movement, making this safety valve irritating and frequently stimulants are taken in order to override it – 'I'll have another cup of coffee / bar of chocolate to keep me going."

If all of this is happening, the person with M.E./C.F.S. is not likely to want to leap out of bed, filled with energy and joy. As the habit of over-breathing grows, then less and less stress causes this reaction and after a time, the body says, 'I can't adapt any more right now. STOP!' Perhaps before developing M.E./C.F.S. the person had to run a half marathon to feel exhausted, but now walking to the gate creates the same feeling.

Overcome Fatigue

The following are given facts:
- Severe or prolonged stress is debilitating (Tortora 1984).
- Stress causes hyperventilation (Timmons 1994)
- Hyperventilation causes stress (Ley 1994)
- It is easy to maintain chronic hyperventilation (Innocenti 1997).

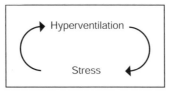

Figure 11:1. The never-ending circle of hyperventilation and stress.

From these facts the conclusion can be drawn that chronic hyperventilation and chronic stress are self-perpetuating, causing both mental and physical exhaustion. To break through this vicious cycle and to allow the body to heal you need to take time out to:

- Restore normal breathing patterns.
- Remove excess stress.
- Develop good dietary habits and drink sufficient water.
- Have adequate sleep.

The most important of all of these is having good breathing habits because breathing directly affects metabolism, heart rate and function, nervous system and the body temperature (Cacioppo 1982). When you breathe correctly, oxygenation is maximised and the body copes better with all kinds of stress. Eating well and drinking sufficient water, removing excess stress, having adequate sleep and doing gentle, no-strain regular exercise as soon as you are able to cope with it will allow the immune system to function more normally and the body to recuperate, restoring energy to your adaptation bank.

'I am very excited about discovering the Buteyko Breathing Techniques because it is totally natural and has given me a lot more energy. To the extent, that it has changed my physical and social lifestyle.' Esther.

References

Cacioppo JT, Petty RE. Perspectives in Cardiovascular Psychophysiology. Guilford Press. New York. 1982.

Fukuda J, Straus SE, Hickie I et al. The chronic fatigue syndrome: a comprehensive approach to its definition and study. International Chronic Fatigue Study Group. Ann Intern Medicine. 1994. 121. pp953-959

Innocenti. DM. Cash's Text Book for Physiotherapists. Chest, Heart and Cardiovascular Conditions. Faber and Faber 1997. p463

Ley R. Behavioural and Psychological Approaches to Breathing Disorders. Ed. B.H. Timmons & R Ley. Plenum. New York. 1994. pp83, 89

Lloyd AR, Hickie I, Boughton CR et al. Prevalence of chronic fatigue syndrome in an Australian population. Medical J Australia. 1990. 153. pp522-528

Selye H. The Stress of Life. Library of Congress Cataloguing in Publication Data. 1984. p 82

Lum LC. Behavioural and Psychological Approaches to Breathing Disorders. Ed. B.H. Timmons & R Ley. Plenum. New York. 1994. p120

Lum, L.C. Respiratory Alkalosis and Hypocarbia The role of carbon dioxide in the body economy. Chest, Heart and Stroke Journal. 1978. 3(4. pp31-34

Timmons BH. Behavioural and Psychological Approaches to Breathing Disorders. Ed. B.H. Timmons & R Ley. Plenum. New York. 1994. p449

Tortora GJ, Anagnostakos NP. Principles of Anatomy and Physiology, Harper & Row, New York. 1984. p429

Chapter 12

Panic or Hyperventilation Attacks

'I was driving my mother-in-law and her sisters in peak hour traffic. It was hot and they were all talking at once. My palms suddenly got sweaty, heart started pounding, I was hot all over, mind was racing and fear gushed up inside me. I really had to fight the urge to stop the car and leap out. I had no idea why I was scared and I was even more worried that they would think I was crazy. It was horrible!' Joy

It is the fear of having a hyperventilation or panic attack like the one above that can create phobias. Knowing that it is irrational to be afraid of driving carefully in traffic does not help, and in fact it is probably not the driving that is so frightening, as much as the fear that the symptoms will recur.

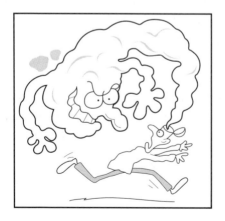

The most common symptoms of hyperventilation attacks are:

- 'Lack of air' sensation
- Chest tightness or pain
- Palpitations, pounding heart, or fast heart rate
- Feeling dizzy, light-headed or faint
- Feeling 'spaced out' or as if you are 'not with it'
- Fear of dying, losing control or going crazy
- Hot all over, sweating especially in the palms or armpits
- Mouth feeling tight and lips may eventually form an "O" shape
- Tense muscles
- Trembling and shaking
- Visual disturbances – blurred or tunnel vision, flashes or shadows before the eyes
- Nausea or stomach upsets
- Numb or tingling sensations in fingers or lips (Fried 1993).

"Hyperventilation as a Cause of Panic Attack" is the title of a research article by Hibbert (1984) and leaves no doubt as to his theory on why these attacks occur. The 'fight or flight' response switches on when danger appears and the surge in breathing, heartbeat, adrenaline and sugar levels occur to maximise the ability to cope with danger. But increasing the breathing rate when there is little need for physical activity, such as when driving a car, is counterproductive because it rapidly lowers carbon dioxide, which is the primary cause of hyperventilation attacks (The Agoraphobic Program Treatment Manual).

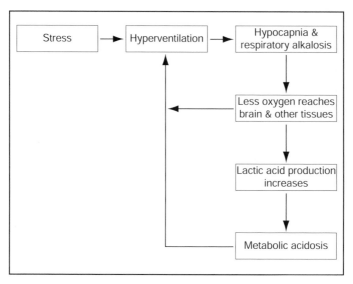

Figure 12:1. Hyperventilation starts the panic attack.

As blood becomes more alkaline, less oxygen is released to tissue cells and more lactic acid is produced, changing the blood pH from alkaline to acidic. To correct this, breathing is intensified.

Due to hypocapnia, smooth muscle throughout the body spasms. That which is wrapped around blood vessels reduces blood flow to the brain and it is estimated that for every one mm Hg reduction in carbon dioxide, the brain receives two per cent less blood flow (Raichle 1972). This is combined with the Bohr effect and means that the brain receives considerably less oxygen than normal, possibly as much as fifty per cent, which is a major stress and can result in feelings of extreme panic (Ley 1994). As the brain becomes concerned about its oxygen supply it stimulates breathing and if hyperventilation is sustained, the person faints. Once this occurs, the brain releases opiates and breathing slows (Danavit-Saubie 1978).

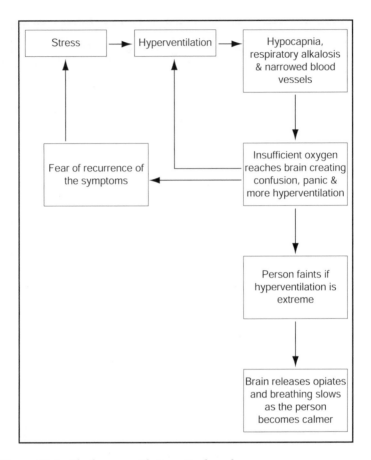

```
┌─────────────┐    ┌──────────────────┐    ┌──────────────────┐
│   Stress    │───▶│ Hyperventilation │───▶│    Hypocapnia,   │
└─────────────┘    └──────────────────┘    │respiratory alkalosis│
       ▲                    ▲               │  & narrowed blood │
       │                    │               │      vessels     │
       │                    │               └──────────────────┘
       │                    │                        │
       │                    │                        ▼
┌──────────────────┐    ┌──────────────────┐
│ Fear of recurrence of│◀─│ Insufficient oxygen│
│   the symptoms    │   │reaches brain creating│
└──────────────────┘   │ confusion, panic & │
                       │ more hyperventilation│
                       └──────────────────┘
                                │
                                ▼
                       ┌──────────────────┐
                       │ Person faints if  │
                       │ hyperventilation is│
                       │     extreme       │
                       └──────────────────┘
                                │
                                ▼
                       ┌──────────────────┐
                       │Brain releases opiates│
                       │and breathing slows │
                       │  as the person    │
                       │  becomes calmer   │
                       └──────────────────┘
```

Figure 12:2. The hyperventilation attack cycle.

While these attacks are frequently called 'Panic Attacks', not everyone feels frightened nor do they all result in fainting. The person may simply notice that the heartbeat is rapid or they feel 'spaced out' with sweaty palms, chest pain or a dry mouth. It is not necessary to breathe exceptionally fast during a hyperventilation attack and while some people do pant, it is common to only see upper chest breathing. The subtlest form of hyperventilation is where the breathing appears normal with intermittent sighs, yawns and gasps (Magarian 1982). The Carbon

Dioxide Syndrome can create a situation where the breathing is marginally faster and/or deeper than is required most of the time, which causes mild apprehension or paranoia, and then it only takes a small stress such as an animated conversation, being in a crowded room or driving the in-laws to produce more noticeable symptoms.

Hyperventilation affects all parts of the body and the actual symptoms a person has as a result largely depend on genetic factors, so it not a reflection of 'weakness' to suffer from hyperventilation attacks. In fact, some researchers believe that they are more commonly found in "A" type personalities (Lum 1978) who are certainly not weak. Instead these people set themselves high goals and are very competitive, wanting to complete a job quicker and better than everyone else.

If the attacks are compounded by focus on a particular symptom, the problem can escalate quickly because recognition of a physical change may be sufficiently stressful to instigate hyperventilation. For example, suppose heart trouble runs in your family and every time you notice that your heart is beating rapidly, you imagine that you are developing the same problem. This fear increases the focus on heartbeat and when it speeds up for even reasonable causes such as during exercise, so will your panic, which in turn speeds up the heart, which increases the fear and so on, until it creates the intense panic that so many people are familiar with.

Feeling frightened for no apparent reason, fearing that you will die, make a complete fool of yourself, or having strange physical symptoms can make you believe that you are going mad. As time goes on, people frequently become more stressed and sometimes they also become depressed. It is important therefore to remember that hyperventilation attacks have a physical cause.

Get Rid of the Panic

Once people identify that they have hyperventilation attacks, they sometimes believe that anxiety is causing the problem. This is not true, as any emotion can initiate an attack and in fact, it would seem that rather than anxiety causing hyperventilation attacks, it is often the other way around (Gardner 1989, Lum 1975 & 1978). First you hyperventilate and then the anxiety develops as a combination of:

- The unpleasant physical sensations of hyperventilation.
- Fear that you will die, or at the very least do something embarrassing.
- Not knowing what is wrong with you but suspecting that it is dangerous.
- Being unable to stop the feelings.

To avoid showing any fear, people learn to bottle up their feelings and put on a composed front. 'I was calm on the outside but screaming on the inside!' is a frequent sentiment of people with this condition. Try to express yourself effectively but tactfully and find ways to let go of the stress as it builds inside you. Physical exercise, meditation, going to a counsellor or just talking to a good friend could be helpful in releasing tension. Tranquilliser medications may be useful in the short term to take the edge off anxiety, but not in the long term because they can be addictive and less effective (Owen 1983) as well as simply masking the symptoms rather than addressing the cause. As hyperventilation further develops and more symptoms appear, either a stronger dose is needed or other forms of treatment may be necessary.

Because the brain requires both oxygen and sugar to function properly, both hyperventilation and low blood sugar can bring on these attacks. Low blood sugar will stimulate the manufacture of adrenaline to enhance sugar production and unfortunately all the other actions of adrenaline, like increased heartbeat and sweating occur as well. It is important therefore to maintain a reasonably constant level of sugar in the blood, which can be achieved by eating small meals several times a day and having some protein at each meal. This is because protein provides a slower and more sustained rise in blood sugar than that formed by carbohydrates (Lum 1994).

Hyperventilation attacks have been jokingly known as 'Designer Jeans Syndrome' when fashion dictates a very slim fit of trousers. This is because clothes that fit tightly around the abdomen encourage upper chest breathing. Babies do not hold their stomach in to look thinner and neither should adults, so the wearing of loose-fitting clothing can be helpful in encouraging a more normal breathing pattern.

A 'lack of air' is a common feeling during a hyperventilation attack, so it is worth remembering that there is a lot more oxygen in the air than is needed by the body. Inhaled air contains approximately 21% oxygen and exhaled air 16%, therefore unless there are *serious* problems with gas exchange it is easy to get plenty of oxygen. The problem starts when there is insufficient carbon dioxide pressure in the bloodstream, which makes it hard to use the oxygen you have already inhaled. The way to ensure that you have adequate levels of carbon dioxide is by keeping your shoulders relaxed and breathing at a moderate pace through your nose. During a hyperventilation attack this could seem impossible to do, so practising while you take part in everyday activities could mean less likelihood of attacks.

Buteyko challenges the theory that deep breathing solves stress-related problems. Blowing up balloons deepens the breathing dramatically yet it certainly doesn't create a sense of relaxation and the worst thing about these attacks is that the hyperventilation, to which you are being driven, is actually causing the symptoms. In an effort to avoid the symptoms, people frequently start to keep away from anything that stimulates breathing such as hot stuffy rooms, caffeine or highly charged emotions. This sounds like good advice, but in reality you are shutting yourself off from life, and in the extreme you could become agoraphobic. Restoring normal breathing patterns so that you are less likely to have an attack in the first place is the best way to overcome this problem.

'Buteyko has lessened the frequency and severity of my panic attacks as well as improved my asthma. I have more energy and greater concentration.' Kerryann

References

Danavit-Saubie M, Champagnat j, Zieglgansberger W. Effect on opiates and metionine-enkephalin on pontint and bulbar respiratory neurones in the cat. Brain Res. 1978. 155. pp55-67

Fried R. The Psychology and Physiology of Breathing. Plenum. New York 1993. pp214-215

Gardner WN, Bass C. Hyperventilation in clinical practice. British J Hospital Medicine. 1989. 41. pp73-81

Hibbert GA. Hyperventilation as a Cause of Panic Attack. Brit Medical Journal. 1984. 288. pp263-264

Ley R. In Behavioural and Psychological Approaches to Breathing Disorders. Ed. B.H. Timmons & R Ley. Plenum. New York. 1994. p87

Lum LC. Behavioural and Psychological Approaches to Breathing Disorders. Ed. B.H. Timmons & R Ley. Plenum. New York. 1994. p119

Lum LC. Hyperventilation: The tip and the iceberg. J Psychosom Res. 1975. 19. pp375-383

Lum LC. Respiratory Alkalosis and Hypocarbia. The roles of carbon dioxide in the body economy. Chest, Heart & Stroke. Winter 1978/79. 3(4). pp31-34

Magarian GJ. Hyperventilation Syndromes: Infrequently Recognized Common Expressions of Anxiety and Stress. Medicine. The Williams and Wilkins Co. 1982. 61 (4). pp219-236

Owen RT, Tyrer P. Benzodiazepine dependence: a review of the evidence. Drugs. 1983. 25. pp385

Raichle ME, Plum E. Hyperventilation and cerebral blood flow. Stroke. 1972. 3. pp566-575

The Agoraphobic Program Treatment Manual. St. Vincent's Hospital, Sydney. 1993. p2

Chapter 13

Stress and Pain Management

'One thing I noticed was that the tension on people's faces lessened as the [Buteyko] course progressed and women who I thought looked old looked several years younger.' Fay

Stress stimulates the breathing and stimulating the breathing increases stress. For example, when experiencing anger it is possible to increase the feeling by breathing faster and deeper, and breathing gently through the nose helps to suppress it. Hidden hyperventilation winds up both the mind and body and is not something that we are aware of, unlike other stress-causing activities such as bereavement or moving house.

The physical symptoms of stress, like feeling exhausted yet not being able to stay asleep, can create uncertainty as to whether the cause is all in the mind or whether an illness is imminent. Few people cope really well with the concept of illness, imagined or otherwise, making it little wonder that the person may become fearful, anxious and irritable or depressed.

The mind is on constant alert when you are stressed and it may start to focus on particular things. In a physically stressful situation, such as an imminent motor vehicle accident, this is useful to see clearly and to make instant decisions. But in hyperventilation-related stress, it can lead to some mental 'tunnel vision' as the perceived source of the problem is focused on. Things may seem to crowd in, and activities or situations become overwhelming. For example being in a room that is too warm, riding in an elevator, having closed windows or being too close to someone can instigate feelings of claustrophobia and even hugging a child or making love can become difficult. The thought, 'I *need* some air!' can be expressed physically by opening a window or metaphorically by walking out of a job or a relationship.

Another well-documented form of stress is Pre-Menstrual Syndrome (PMS). At this time of the menstrual cycle, progesterone is the dominating hormone circulating in a woman's body and one effect of progesterone is to increase the breathing pattern (Sukkar 1993). It is little wonder then that women who also suffer from the Carbon Dioxide Syndrome have an increase in symptoms when their own body is causing them breathe more air each minute.

When a person is stressed, it affects the entire family and all close associates. At this time the person usually believes that they are not the one with the problem, and as others struggle to cope with fluctuating moods and apparent irrationality, there will be negative feedback that contributes to the build-up of stress. Typically people attempt to cope with stress by cleaning the ashtrays while the Titanic sinks, so to speak. They may:

- Make lifestyle changes - move house, get divorced, change jobs or try new diets.
- Opt out of society and refuse to conform.
- Drink alcohol excessively or take drugs.
- Feel the need to gamble or to compete and win at all costs.
- Constantly collect new toys, such as cars, furniture, babies and clothes.
- Become totally absorbed with a new interest.

All of the above can temporarily give a 'high' or distraction from the real problem and make the person feel better about their current situation or their self-image, but long-term it is not helping to promote good physical or mental health.

Reduce Stress

Since chronic stress and chronic hyperventilation go hand in hand and feed each other, to break the vicious cycle you need to tackle the problem of stress management from different angles, which could include:

- Take time out to do activities that you enjoy doing.
- Try to think more along the lines of, "If I broke my leg and wasn't be able to do this task, would it *really* matter?"
- Do not breathe deeply when you get upset.
- Watch or read comedies to get some laughter into your life.
- Get regular physical exercise, such as walking, dancing, running, swimming or playing squash.
- Have a healthy diet, but remember that a little indulgence from time to time does little harm.
- Use fewer stimulants such as coffee and tobacco.
- Have regular massages – if money is a problem then swap with a friend because even a less than perfect massage is better than no massage for reducing stress.
- Get a pet or spend time with other people's pets.
- Talk to someone about your problems; this could be your best friend, a stranger on the bus or a professional counsellor, psychologist or psychiatrist.
- Alcohol and drugs are potential poisons, not to mention sometimes illegal, so if you must use them, be cautious as they can cause more problems than they solve.

When you increase your breathing pattern, you are telling your brain that it needs to prepare the body for possible danger. When properly applied, the Buteyko Method helps to reduce stress levels because it deliberately reverses this process. Now you start to tell your brain, 'It's OK. I'm safe.' and the brain stops sending messages all around the body to prepare for an attack.

The theory of Buteyko is not new. It is possible to read about how oxygen is the fuel and carbon dioxide the regulator of the human body in any physiology textbook. The Bohr effect has been written up in these same textbooks for approximately one hundred years. It has long been noted that an abnormally low pressure of carbon dioxide in the bloodstream seriously affects the workings of all metabolic processes in the body; in fact American Doctor, Yandell Henderson, killed dogs by quickly lowering their carbon dioxide pressure in 1908. Even the application of Buteyko-type breathing is not new: over two thousand years ago Lao-Tzu, who practised Tibetan medicine, is reported as saying , "The perfect man breathes as if he is not breathing."

Being 'stressed to the max' makes it difficult to think properly or to realise that all anyone really needs apart from the basic shelter and food, is people you care about and who care about you. Modern people still live in a body of ancient design that was not intended to cope with prolonged stress such as driving a motor car at one hundred kilometres an hour or sitting at a computer every day. Practising the Buteyko Method enables you to take much of the stress out of life by changing your breathing pattern; in other words, you stop cleaning the ashtrays.

'Buteyko has taken huge stress out of my life. I am grateful for the improvement in the quality of my life which in turn helps my family and career.' John

Pain

Pain is a common source of stress, and pain and breathing are closely connected. A sudden stab of pain temporarily stops the breathing, whereas continued pain increases it. Perhaps this is because stimulation of the breathing pattern seems to have an analgesic effect (Glynn 1981). People who walk on fire or pierce their skin with needles during religious ceremonies usually prepare for these events by hyperventilating and they do not appear to suffer any pain (Lum 1981).

While hyperventilation can be used to numb pain, conversely some pain may be result of hyperventilation. British cardiologist, Peter Nixon, suggests that 80% of people suffering from angina are primarily suffering from hyperventilation (Perera 1988). Angina pain is a result of inadequate oxygen supplies reaching the heart, causing a build-up of lactic acid in this area and hyperventilation could easily cause this to happen. Chest pain unrelated to angina can also be caused by hyperventilation and could be due to muscle tension or overuse of the chest muscles. Changing the posture and breathing pattern often relieves it.

Lack of oxygen can also create pain or inflammation in other parts of the body, which may be relieved when the breathing pattern is decreased. People often predict weather changes by their 'rheumatics' and heat, humidity or a sudden drop in barometric pressure can trigger hyperventilation (Lum 1994).

Migraine is another painful experience that is linked by some researchers to hyperventilation. It is thought that migraine headaches are caused by spasm of arteries within the brain. This causes a lack of oxygen to these areas and pain results. If the person already has a weakness in the circulatory system then hyperventilation may be a contributing factor, as it is known to cause spasm of arteries and alkalosis, both of which lessen the delivery of oxygen (Fried 1993).

Manage Pain

Pain relief medications are readily available, though their long-term or overuse is not recommended. All medications are filtered through either the kidneys or liver, so taking any drugs places some pressure on these organs. Surgery may also be an option for some people, depending on the source of the problem.

There are also a number of non-drug or surgical treatments, which may help to alleviate pain and these include:

Acupuncture or acupressure	Alexander techniques
Aromatherapy	Chiropractics
Cold packs	Feldenkrais techniques
Hot baths or packs	Hypnotism
Laughter	Massage
Owning a pet	Physiotherapy
Tai Chi	Yoga

Relieving chronic pain, whether through breathing or other modalities is a good way to release tension and to also restore better health.

'I have lost the aching feeling in my feet. Before Buteyko, the pain in my feet was crippling when I woke up.' Lesley

References

Fried R. The Psychology and Physiology of Breathing. Plenum Press. New York 1993. p208.

Glynn CJ, Lloyd, JW, Folkhard S. Ventilatory response to intractable pain. Pain. 1981. 11. pp201-211

Henderson Y. Acapnia and Shock, American. J. of Physiology 1908. 21. pp125-156

Lum LC. Behavioural and Psychological Approaches to Breathing Disorders. Ed. B.H. Timmons & R Ley. Plenum. New York. 1994

Lum LC. Hyperventilation and the anxiety state. Journal of the Royal Society of Medicine. 1981. 74. pp1– 4

Perera J. Hazards of Heavy Breathing. New Scientist. December 1988. pp46–48

Sukkar MY, El-Munshid HA & Ardawi. Concise Human Physiology. Blackwell Scientific Publications. Oxford. 1993. p342

Chapter 14

Lung Damage

Having asthma is not something that anyone would like to have and neither is bronchitis, but having one or the other is more manageable than the two combined. When one condition runs into the other, instead of having slight symptoms of one condition the overall symptoms are a lot worse. For example, with asthma there are periods where the airways are narrowed and it is difficult to get air out of the lungs and with bronchitis there are extreme amounts of mucus with an almost constant cough. When these conditions combine, it is not only difficult to move air out of the lungs, but even harder to remove the excessive mucus.

As the conditions worsen they develop into what is called C.O.P.D., C.O.R.D. or C.O.A.D. (Chronic Obstructive Pulmonary/Respiratory/Airway Disease). Conditions that fall into this category include emphysema, chronic bronchitis, bronchiectasis and chronic, severe asthma. C.O.P.D. is progressive, with damage to the lungs getting worse over time and leading to a more restricted lifestyle.

The lungs are warm and damp, making them an ideal breeding ground for bacteria and fungi that release toxic chemicals that do permanent damage. If the person has a depressed immune system then this is more of a problem. However, the nose has a wonderful filtration system and when it is used for breathing, the lungs remain virtually sterile. Lungs also have a self-cleaning system that consists of a mucus blanket sitting on tiny hair-like

165

structures called cilia in the airways. Cilia act like an escalator or conveyor belt, moving the mucus blanket and any dust, germs and other debris out of the lungs at a rate of approximately one centimetre each minute (Guyton 1982). (Figure 14.1.) Unfortunately this system is fragile and easily damaged.

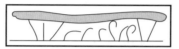

Figure 14:1. Cilia and the mucus blanket help to clean and protect the airways.

Most people with damaged lungs have smoked cigarettes, been exposed to lots of irritants such as dust, toxic fumes and pollution or have suffered multiple chest infections, all of which establish prolonged inflammation (Crompton 1987). Chronic inflammation scars the airway walls and where there is scarring, cilia disappear and the 'escalator' cannot move the mucus blanket properly. As mucus pools in the damaged areas, it becomes prone to infection, and to compound the problem, mucus thickens to prevent infection spreading and becomes even more difficult to shift (Lumb 2000). Scarring also makes the airways lose tone and elasticity, causing 'floppy airways'.

It is now common knowledge that smoking is not a healthy pastime, but people who have damaged their lungs in this way were not always aware of this when they started. In fact, they may even have been encouraged to take up smoking to reduce stress. Today they are more likely to be linked to depression and pain, creating stress instead of alleviating it (Hough 1997).[5]

Only a few decades ago, there were almost no limits on pollution emissions into the atmosphere and people worked without protection in environments that were dusty or filled with fumes. Breathing through the mouth or smoking in these surroundings draws more irritants directly into the lungs where they do damage. Mouth breathing could be a common factor with many chronic lung diseases because according to Gardner et al (1990), it is possible that all respiratory diseases may have hyperventilation and hypocapnia as a feature in their early stages.

Chest infections damage the lungs and are potential killers, so the body does its best to keep out germs by using inflammation, heat and an army of chemicals to prevent their entry, contain them, or to kill them off. Alternatively, they are violently expelled by sneezing or coughing. However, when the invaders are more than can be handled, the person gets sick. Constant hyperventilation suppresses the immune system (Timmons 1994), and increases the likelihood of sickness and infection.

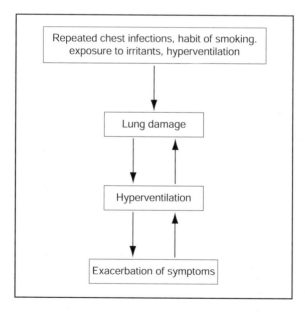

Figure 14:2. Many things cause lung damage and the damage itself perpetuates the problem.

Emphysema

Alveoli are vital for good health as it is here that external gas exchange takes place. With emphysema the alveoli are damaged (Figure 14.4) and this makes it harder for oxygen to reach the bloodstream and ultimately tissue cells. Consequently the heart works harder and the whole body suffers as a result of receiving less oxygen.

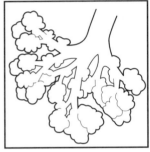

Figure 14:3. Healthy alveoli.   *Figure 14:4. Emphysematous*
alveoli.

Like balloons, lungs are made of an elastic-type substance that can be blown up and let down many times. After a balloon has been blown up and let down several times it doesn't shrink back to its original size. This is particularly true of balloons that are over-inflated. The lungs are made of much better material than balloons but they also suffer when blown up repeatedly under great pressure.

Activities such as glass blowing, playing the saxophone or repeated coughing, which induce strenuous breathing, may lead to emphysema because excess pressure in the alveoli can rupture the alveolar walls and many alveoli merge into one sac instead of lots of tiny sacs (Guyton 1982, Medical Encyclopaedia & St. John's Mercy web sites). Because the lungs are less elastic, they become permanently inflated and the chest also has to increase in size to accommodate them.

Chronic Bronchitis

In chronic bronchitis the mucus cells in the airways are both enlarged and more numerous than average and consequently the mucus production is greatly increased. Cilia become damaged, which makes the clearance of mucus more difficult and increases the risk of infection (Lumb 2000).

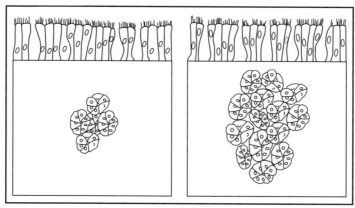

Figure 14:5. A comparison of normal mucus producing cells (left) and those in Chronic Bronchitis (right).

The associated chronic inflammation narrows airways, limits airflow and sets up a pattern of wheezing, coughing and repeated chest infections. These are mild to begin with, and the person can have chronic bronchitis for years before it becomes a major problem. Red blood cell production increases in an effort to compensate for less oxygen reaching the bloodstream, which thickens the blood and makes the heart work harder, raising blood pressure, creating headaches and ultimately making oxygen delivery even more difficult (Hough 1997).

Bronchiectasis

Bronchiectasis is a condition where there is an abnormal dilation and distortion of airways, which is commonly caused by a foreign body lodged in the airways, or a severe viral chest infection. Instead of being smooth tubes, the airways become corrugated. When it is not possible to get sufficient air, the person typically increases the speed of breathing to compensate, but rapid breathing is difficult due to the damage caused by bronchiectasis, which can lead to poor oxygenation and fatigue.

Because of the size, damage, loss of cilia and corrugations, mucus pools in the airways and leads to chronic bacterial infection. Vast quantities of horrible smelling and discoloured phlegm are produced and even though coughing is less effective due to the damaged airways, it is still common for the person to cough up more than a cup of mucus every day during 'postural drainage'. Postural drainage means to lie in a position where the head and chest are lower than the rest of the body. Using gravity and coughing, excess mucus is removed from the lungs.

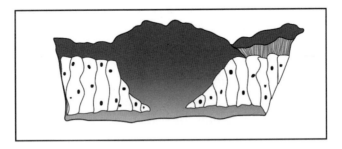

Figure 14:6. Mucus and pus build up where the lungs are damaged and encourage chronic infections.

Dealing With C.O.P.D.

There are a number of things that will immediately make a difference to a person with chronic lung disease:

- Stop smoking
- Keep your shoulders relaxed
- Control your coughing
- Pace yourself so that you do not get puffed
- Exercise regularly but without stress
- Breathe through your nose all the time
- Look after your health
- Use the Buteyko Institute Method.

Stop Smoking

Deliberately filling your lungs with tar and other toxins is suicide in slow motion and apart from the risk of lung cancer or gangrene you face the prospect of lengthy suffocation from emphysema or chronic bronchitis. If you still smoke, do yourself a HUGE favour and STOP!! If you cannot do this alone, then enter one of the many programmes that help people to quit smoking.

Relax Your Shoulders

Having a chronic lung disease is particularly stressful and consequently muscle tension is high, which is particularly noted in the neck and shoulders but can be found throughout the whole body. Having a regular massage or practising a muscle relaxation sequence can be helpful to release muscle tension.

Like balloons, lungs are easier to get air into when they are half inflated, rather than completely flat or when they are already filled with air. Gulping air through your mouth and using your upper chest encourages mucus production and narrowing of the airways, which traps air in the lungs and leads to over-inflation.

Try hunching your shoulders while you breathe. Notice how much effort it takes, especially when you exhale. Now consciously drop your shoulders and feel how easily the air moves in and out of your body. With your shoulders relaxed, you are also more likely to use the diaphragm, which is the most efficient muscle for breathing. When the work of breathing is easier, you need less oxygen to accomplish it.

Control the Coughing

Coughing very hard is not beneficial because it can limit airflow, lower the pressure of oxygen in the bloodstream and cause the heart rhythm to become disturbed as well as causing muscle pains and even occasionally breaking ribs (Pryor 1998). On the other hand, the cough reflex can save lives by removing foreign particles from the throat and lungs, so the type of coughing that you do may be important. As mucus is swept up the airways it piles up in areas where there are no cilia and when it eventually spills over onto the next healthy section, a coughing spasm is initiated. Coughing softly with a closed mouth helps to move mucus which may become infected if it sits in one spot, but does not put the lungs under as much pressure as a loud, hard and hacking cough.

Remember:
- Mucus is a natural secretion that is required by the lungs for normal function so do not try to cough it *all* up.
- Breathing through your nose will lessen mucus production and stop it from drying out.
- Drinking plenty of water or other fluid that is not a diuretic will help to keep mucus moving, which will assist the cilia to eliminate the excess.

Go at Your Own Pace

Only approximately one tenth of the total lung capacity is required for sufficient gas exchange while resting (Coope 1948), but this can greatly increase while exercising, so if your lung capacity is already diminished, then go more slowly.

The fear of being breathless and not being able to catch your breath is possibly worse than actually being breathless. Since panic heightens the need for oxygen, try to stay calm in all situations. Anyone can get breathless; children get breathless while running around with their friends but instead of worrying about it, they sit down until they have recovered. You can try the same idea by slowing down or stopping when you *begin* to get puffed, which will mean a faster recovery and less breathlessness in the long run. It might take an hour to do something that used to take forty-five minutes, but very often this is of little importance.

Breathe through your nose all the time, and take special notice that you do this while getting out of a chair, getting dressed or having a shower. When you already feel breathless, breathing through your nose will not feel like the right thing to do, but recovery is faster than when you breathe through your mouth.

Keep Physically Fit

Some breathlessness may simply be due to lack of physical fitness or being overweight. Everyone should do regular exercise and when you have damaged lungs, staying fit is of particular importance. It is easy to get into the cycle of doing less exercise because it makes you breathless.

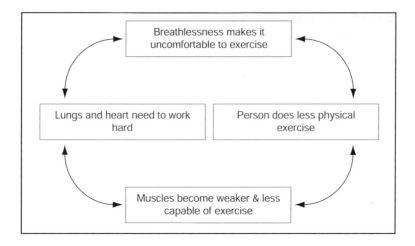

Figure 14:7. Doing little or no exercise creates a vicious circle.

But while it is essential for a person with lung damage to keep fit, the level of exercise should not cause excessive breathlessness as this is unproductive and leads to more hyperventilation. Work within your capabilities and if walking to the letter box is all you can do today, then that is all you do. As you improve, then extend the distance or go a little faster. Always make your pace *fit* your breathing pattern and *not* the other way around. Should you accidentally over-exercise it is easy to reach the point where you want to breathe in before you have finished breathing out. If this occurs, slow down your pace or sit down and remember to keep your shoulders relaxed while still continuing to breathe through your nose.

Breathe Moderately

Breathing excessively fast, especially through your mouth, only irritates airways and makes it more difficult to use the oxygen that you have already inhaled. Breathing through your nose filters out germs (fewer chest infections) and irritants (less inflammation and mucus production). It moistens and warms the air you breathe (less dry, sticky mucus) and your lungs will work more efficiently (less breathlessness and strain on the heart), which is exactly what you want.

The hyperventilation associated with C.O.P.D. may be created by the lack of oxygen reaching the bloodstream, but frequently it is compounded by a panic component because being breathless can be frightening. However, rising panic increases the sense of breathlessness and can create a vicious circle, so it is important to gain control of excessive breathing. Because the gas exchange in the lungs is impaired and the work of breathing is excessive, there may be an excess of carbon dioxide in the blood but there will still be less than normal within the lungs while hyperventilation is maintained. It is believed by promoters of Buteyko that the low pressure of carbon dioxide in the lungs contributes to the spasm of smooth muscle, swelling of the airways and excessive mucus production found in these conditions. Controlling the breathing by breathing through your nose will help to reverse the loss of carbon dioxide in the lungs and will go a long way towards improving the situation.

Look After Your Health

When animals are sick, they usually eat minimally, drink lots of water, find a quiet place and rest. Instead of taking the 'soldier on' attitude, you can try helping yourself in a similar fashion so that the immune system is more effective in promoting good health. Recall the number of times you have felt that you were coming down with a cold and instead of going out, you had a warm drink, put your feet up and watched television or read a book all evening and in the morning you were perfectly fine.

The Buteyko Institute Method

By practising Buteyko exercises the hyperventilation that is constantly irritating the airways; causing loss of carbon dioxide in the lungs, if not the bloodstream, as well as contributing to breathlessness and panic, begins to slow down. However, it is highly unlikely that the Buteyko Method will reverse the damage that has already been done and sudden bursts of activity, like rushing to answer the phone, will more than likely still give some problems. However, people with damaged lungs who practise the exercises regularly are pleasantly surprised to find that they:

- Are less breathless
- Produce less mucus
- Have less airway inflammation
- Sleep more soundly
- Require less medication
- Have less tension and panic
- Are able to exercise more easily.

'The improvement in my overall health has been dramatic. I rate my health as pre- and post-Buteyko. Pre-Buteyko meant colds, coughs, and bronchitis every 6 weeks. Post-Buteyko means increased energy, lack of dizziness, and coughs and colds only 2-3 times a year.' Clare

Yandell Henderson and his colleagues demonstrated that by applying air that contained 8% carbon dioxide to dogs with pneumonia for 12 – 24 hours, they were cured of pneumonia (Henderson 1940). Henderson and Howard Haggard then went on to develop a special tent that was used for treatment of humans with pneumonia. Applying the Buteyko Institute Method may not be as effective as this, but on the whole it means that you are likely to have fewer chest infections.

Like most things, you only get out of Buteyko what you put into it and following the guidance of your teacher and being persistent with the exercises is the key. People with damaged lungs need to practise the Buteyko exercises daily to maintain their progress and while it is unlikely that the damage will be reversed, the progression of C.O.P.D. may be slowed and as your breathing improves, life will seem more worthwhile.

'Although I have emphysema I have found a tremendous difference in my breathlessness. Now it's just mild in the mornings. My doctor and chemist are amazed at the difference; they can't believe it improved so quickly in the past three months. I personally am enjoying each day, instead of dreading the dawning of a new day.' Helen

References

Coope Robert. Diseases of the Chest. E & S Livingstone. 1948. p8

Crompton GK. Greening AP. Drug Use in Respiratory Disease. Williams & Wilkins. Sydney. 1987. p136

Gardner WN, Green SE, Ford TA. Measurement of end-tidal PCO_2 during lung function measurement. American Review of Respiratory Diseases. 1990. 141. p308

Guyton. AC. Human Physiology and Mechanisms of Disease. W.B. Saunders Co. Philadelphia. 1982. pp301, 325-327

Henderson Y. Cyclopedia of Medicine. 1940

Hough A. Physiotherapy in Respiratory Care. Stanley Thornes Ltd. London.1997. pp 1, 2, 17, 53

http://www.stjohnsmercy.org/mmg/mmghealthinfo/adults/respiratoryconditions/COPD.asp

http://www.medicplanet.com/MP_article/internal_reference/Emphysema

Lumb AB. Nunn's Applied Respiratory Physiology. Reed. London. 2000. pp23, 26

Pryor JA, Webber BA. Physiotherapy for Respiratory and Cardiac Problem. Churchill Livingstone. London. 1998. pp239-240

Timmons BH. Behavioural and Psychological Approaches to Breathing Disorders. Ed. B.H. Timmons & R Ley. Plenum. New York. 1994. p263

Chapter 15

Urinary and Digestive Systems

There is a lot of smooth muscle in the digestive tract as well as mast cells that release histamine. Kidneys also play a vital role in maintaining the ionic balance, so it is little wonder that people with the Carbon Dioxide Syndrome notice problems with these parts of their body.

A frequent complaint of people with the Carbon Dioxide Syndrome is the increased need to urinate. They wake up two or three times a night to go to the bathroom, or they cannot sit through a meeting. This frequent urge to urinate can be for a number of reasons:

- When the fight or flight response is triggered, blood pressure rises quickly. To regulate blood pressure an enormous amount of urine is produced and rapidly needs to be voided.
- Hidden hyperventilation causes smooth muscle in the bladder wall to spasm, with extra discomfort.
- When hidden hyperventilation has become the norm, the kidneys are required to dump bicarbonates regularly to balance the pH. This means an increasing need to urinate.
- The fear that it may be necessary to use the toilet and the opportunity will not easily arise contributes to the problem by creating more stress.

People with dysfunctional breathing also often have digestive problems, like producing too much gas, bloating, constipation, diarrhoea, indigestion, ulcers, and nausea. Hyperventilation shuts down digestion and hypocapnia stimulates mast cells in the gut to release more histamine, contributing to inflammation and spasm of smooth muscle. Instead of food being pulsed smoothly through the body, its passage slows or speeds up as the smooth muscle wrapped around the digestive tract contracts and relaxes with the surging carbon dioxide pressure.

Irritable bowel syndrome is caused by abnormal muscle contractions in the digestive tract (Tortora 1984) and is arguably worse than a 'weak' bladder. Not only is the intermittent diarrhoea a nuisance and embarrassing but the constipation is painful. Vomiting or having several bowel movements a day can lead to malnutrition and pH disturbances.

Improve Gastro-Intestinal Disorders

It would seem that the body responds favourably to some basic rules:

- Eat moderate amounts of food regularly throughout the day and avoid irritants
- Drink adequate amounts of water
- Take regular physical exercise
- Breathe less.

Avoiding known irritants such as excessive amounts of caffeine, alcohol and very spicy or sugary foods may help to lessen bloating and general irritation of both the bowel and bladder. Eating a balanced diet with several small meals a day, rather than two or three large meals is useful, as is including adequate quantities of fibre.

Drink plenty of water during the day and early evening, but avoid having several glasses just before bedtime, and this may improve the likelihood of sleeping through the night instead of waking up to go to the bathroom.

Taking regular exercise that is manageable and does not aggravate the breathing is another way to help the body to work more efficiently. See chapter ten for more information on developing an exercise programme.

Being able to switch off hidden hyperventilation is a big help in settling down the digestive tract, and as breathing becomes more normal the things that caused you irritation rapidly become less of a problem. This makes it possible to have the occasional alcoholic drink or chocolate milk shake without the unwanted effects that these things currently cause.

'Life for 4-year-old Stella before Buteyko: constant stomach cramps, vomiting, constant urinating (20 times a day), fretfulness, grizzling, coughing, waking up to 5 times a night and the dreaded asthma requiring hospitalisation on occasions. Buteyko has given Stella a real life. The returns on my investment in Buteyko have been beyond all my expectations.' Anne (Stella's mother)

References
Tortora GJ, Anagnostakos NP. Principles of Anatomy and Physiology, Harper & Row, New York. 1984. p625

Chapter 16

High Blood Pressure

High blood pressure or hypertension is a condition that has become almost epidemic in today's world. It kills more people than cancer and does this literally by strangling the body. Arteries narrow and the brain, heart and limbs receive insufficient blood that is carrying their vital oxygen and nutrients.

Blood flows from the heart where blood pressure is highest to other parts of the body where the pressure is lower. The pressure is the force that the heart exerts on the blood to move it around the body and is primarily determined by how much blood is pumped each time out of the heart into the main artery (aorta). Blood presses against the walls of the blood vessels, which stretch and contract to help push the blood around. If there is an increase in blood volume due to fluid retention, or the blood vessels are narrow and do not stretch properly, then the pressure rises because the heart has to work harder to move the blood around. This is called 'high blood pressure' or 'hypertension'.

When blood pressure is taken, two numbers are noted, 120 / 80 for example. Like the pressure of gases, these figures refer to millimetres of mercury (mm Hg) and the amount of mercury the pressure would support. The first number refers to the systolic pressure, which is when the left ventricle of the heart contracts and shoots oxygenated blood into the aorta. After this, the heart has a tiny rest and the pressure drops, giving the second number (diastolic pressure).

Blood pressure is typically considered high when the numbers are at least 140 / 90 when a person is not yet forty years old and 160/95 once the person is older than this. 'Low' blood pressure or 'hypotension' is declared when the readings are approximately 100 / 70 or less and generally refers to a sudden drop in pressure.

If blood pressure were to be taken continuously it would be noted that it constantly changes, because as blood pressure rises the body automatically takes actions to lower it, and when it becomes too low the pressure is raised. This way blood pressure stays within the healthy range. The following factors regulate blood pressure:

- The kidneys play a primary role by controlling the volume of blood and also by excreting or restoring minerals to the bloodstream.
- The tension of smooth muscle that is wrapped around blood vessels – spasmed smooth muscle raises blood pressure.
- The thickness of the blood, for example when blood is thickened it moves more slowly than when it is very fluid and the pressure increases to push it around.
- Irregularities in the surface of the blood vessels tend to slow down the flow, which increases the pressure (Guyton 1982).

Factors that create a rise in blood pressure include: diseased kidneys; stress; the production of acetylcholine by the brain; snoring and sleep apnoea; exercise; hyperventilation; an increase in the volume of blood; lack of oxygen in the tissues; hardened arteries, and some medications. Cholesterol, which is a fatty substance that is absorbed from foods and also manufactured by the liver to make bile acids and steroid hormones, contributes to hypertension by sticking to the arterial walls and preventing them from being as pliable as they should be ('hardening of the arteries'). This makes the arteries more likely to rupture rather than stretching and the roughness of the deposits on the walls can cause blood clots to develop.

Factors that cause blood pressure to drop include: going into shock; diabetes; Addison's disease; alcoholism; the aftermath of exercise; hyperventilation; being in the sauna; standing up too suddenly; the loss of blood, and some medications.

There are two types of hypertension: primary and secondary. Secondary hypertension is usually caused by kidney disease, atherosclerosis or too much of the hormone aldosterone which is released by the adrenal glands. This type of hypertension accounts for approximately 15% of sufferers. The other 85% have primary hypertension and modern medicine can find no organic cause for this (Tortora 1984).

Hyperventilation-Related Hypertension

Hyperventilation elevates blood pressure, which in the short term may be beneficial while running to safety or defending yourself, as it rushes blood to areas of the body that rapidly need it. However, the bad habit of hidden hyperventilation can also raise blood pressure and this is normally long term. People with the Carbon Dioxide Syndrome and a genetic tendency to hypertension no doubt have a greater problem with this, than a person with a genetic tendency towards asthma for example. If a person visits a doctor for hypertension and begins drug treatment for it, but does nothing about the hidden hyperventilation, then the hyperventilation will only get worse and either the blood pressure will creep higher, requiring extra medication, or other symptoms of hyperventilation develop.

The Risks

Uncontrolled hypertension can cause considerable damage to the heart, kidneys and brain (Tortora 1984). For example, when the heart has to work harder due to increased blood pressure it becomes larger, which means that it requires more oxygen to function properly. If this need is not met, then the person is more likely to develop angina and the risk of heart attack is greater. The tiny blood vessels in the brain are more likely to tear if too much pressure is placed on them, which means they bleed into the brain, causing a cerebral vascular accident or what is commonly caused a stroke. The kidneys are also at greater risk because the constant high pressure of the blood thickens the walls of the tiny blood vessels feeding the kidneys and reduces the supply of oxygen, eventually damaging the kidneys. Atherosclerosis or hardening of the arteries, which contributes to high blood pressure, is made worse by high blood pressure, thus creating a vicious circle.

Improve Hypertension

Regular moderate exercise is essential in maintaining good health and it is also a good way to assist in weight loss, which alone may help to reduce blood pressure. To make even more improvement, it may be worth consulting a dietician or nutritionist to determine a suitable diet that will help you to maintain a healthy weight and to also eliminate excessive cholesterol intake.

Because nicotine narrows blood vessels and contributes to the problem of hypertension, this is as good a reason as any to stop smoking and one that will do the rest of your body a favour at the same time.

Using too much salt or sodium is something that people with hypertension are usually warned about because there is a link between sodium and hypertension, but the case for eliminating all salt is not yet certain. While having an excess of sodium is not good for anyone, a deficiency can mean an increase in the low density lipoproteins that carry cholesterol to the arteries. Calcium channel blockers, which are commonly used to treat hypertension, and ineffective when the person is on a low-salt diet (Youngsen 1997). Since this issue is unresolved, perhaps having the correct balance of minerals in the body is healthier than having an excess or deficiency.

Studies show that by slowing the breathing down to ten breaths per minute for fifteen minutes at a time, three to four times a week improves hypertension when a special device is used (Grossman 2001, Schein 2001). The Buteyko Institute Method is not about deliberately slowing your breathing down in this manner. However, many people with hypertension have experienced great improvement in their control over this condition simply by practising the Buteyko exercises.

References

Fried R. The hyperventilation Syndrome Research and Clinical Treatment. The John Hopkins University Press. 1987. pp27 - 30, 42

Grossman E, Grossman A, Schein MH, Zimlichman R, Gavish B. 'Breathing-control lowers blood pressure. J Human Hypertension. 2001;15(4):263–269

Guyton. AC. Human Physiology and Mechanisms of Disease. W.B. Saunders Co. Philadelphia. 1982. pp161-168

Schein M, Gavish B, Herz M et al. 'Treating hypertension with a device that slows and regulizes breathing: a randomised double-blind controlled study.' J Human Hypertension. 2001. 15(4). pp271-278

Tortora GJ, Anagnostakos NP. Principles of Anatomy and Physiology, Harper & Row, New York. 1984. p515

Youngsen R. The People's Medical Society. Blood Pressure: Questions You Have – Answers You Want. Thorsons. London. 1997. p28

Chapter 17

Diabetes

There is a common misconception that the eating of too many sweets causes diabetes, but in actual fact it is caused by a disturbance in the metabolism of carbohydrates.

There are two types of diabetes – diabetes insipidus and diabetes mellitus. Diabetes insipidus is caused when the body does not produce enough antidiuretic hormones, which means that urination is excessive, which produces a huge thirst. By taking adequate antidiuretic hormone the condition is usually managed successfully. Diabetes mellitus occurs when an excessive amount of sugar is found in the blood and urine. There is also an excessive thirst, increased need to urinate and excessive eating habits, when it is uncontrolled. More than 90% of the people with diabetes mellitus have what is called 'adult-onset'. They do not develop the condition until they are over forty and they are frequently overweight to start with (Tortora 1984).

Insulin is a hormone whose primary job is to lower sugar levels in the blood by making cells accept the sugar. The amount of insulin that is secreted into the bloodstream fluctuates and directly correlates with the level of sugar found there. As well as increasing sugar levels, a decrease in sodium also simulates insulin production (Youngsen 1997). Even though salt was considered so valuable two thousand years ago that Roman soldiers in England were sometimes paid in salt (the word salary comes from 'salt'), many people today are on reduced salt diets. Perhaps this is a contributing factor to the increase in diabetes.

People with adult-onset diabetes usually have either adequate levels or an oversupply of insulin, yet they still do not cope well with the excess of sugar. This form of diabetes is generally controlled by changes in diet and exercise. Juvenile-onset diabetes is a condition that usually develops before the person is twenty years old. These people have an immune reaction that prevents their ability to manufacture insulin, so they require insulin on a regular or continual basis. While the causes of the two types of diabetes are different, the effects and therefore the management can be quite similar. Often this condition is triggered by a major stress such as a viral infection like measles or mumps (Tortora 1984) or the onset of adolescence.

Does Metabolic Acidosis Cause Respiratory Alkalosis?

Metabolic acidosis and alkalosis are abnormalities in body fluid pH that are not caused by breathing incorrectly, but by disturbances in metabolism. For example, excessive vomiting can result in metabolic alkalosis. People with diabetes mellitus have metabolic acidosis and to compensate for this, they hyperventilate to create respiratory alkalosis (Fried 1987). When the metabolism increases, so does the production of carbon dioxide, which has the immediate effect of stimulating breathing to prevent the pH from getting too low. Unfortunately, altering the breathing will not completely correct the pH because as the pH becomes more tolerable, the drive to breathe is lessened, though not completely restored to normal. Now the situation may occur where the pH is slightly more acidic than it should be, and there is a constant need to compensate with hidden hyperventilation, or the kidneys will have to work harder to excrete hydrogen ions.

According to the Buteyko theory, it could also work the other way around when the breathing is increased during prolonged stress, maintaining respiratory alkalosis and causing the body to compensate with metabolic acidosis. Hidden hyperventilation can be maintained for a prolonged period but there are numerous bodily changes, which include:

- Both carbon dioxide pressure and the number of hydrogen ions become lower because of the increased breathing pattern
- Sugar levels are boosted
- Insulin levels increase to deal with the extra sugar
- The break down of protein and fats is speeded up to provide energy
- Digestion slows down
- Urination increases.

It is possible that both Professor Buteyko and conventional medicine are both correct and some people have metabolic acidosis first, while others have respiratory alkalosis. The important thing to consider is whether changing your breathing can correct the situation. In the case of adult-onset diabetes that is not managed by drugs, changing the breathing could be the one thing that you have not yet tried to manage your condition. On the other hand, if conventional medicine is correct and hyperventilation is necessary to counteract the metabolic acidosis that diabetes causes, then changing your breathing patterns could make your condition markedly worse.

Reducing the Dangers

Guthrie, Moeller and Guthrie (1983) demonstrated that by undergoing relaxation training, the diabetic patients in their study became less insulin dependent. They surmised that this

189

was because when stress is reduced, so is blood glucose, which therefore lessens the need for insulin. If you take insulin to control your diabetes then it is imperative that you do not undertake learning the Buteyko Method without the assistance of an experienced Buteyko practitioner and the support of your doctor. Your condition must be checked regularly and extreme care taken to adjust your insulin so that your condition remains stable, because not doing this could be disastrous to your health and safety.

People with diabetes are prone to other health disorders such as problems with the nervous system, circulation, heart disease, kidney failure, cataracts, blindness and infections, so maintaining a healthy lifestyle is most important.

Muscle-wasting and weight loss is a probability if insulin is not kept at the right balance, so eating well, with the right kinds of foods at the right time, will help to not only keep the sugar levels steady but to also maintain a healthy weight. Sugar levels in the blood and urine need to be checked regularly so that adjustments can be made when necessary to diet and/or insulin levels. Electrolyte disturbances are likely to occur in diabetics and there is a special problem with maintaining sufficient potassium levels, which is vital to normal heart function. This is another important consideration for management of the diet.

Regular exercise is important with all people, and diabetics are no exception. However, since healing is delayed, there is a tendency to get infections and diabetics are more prone to gangrene than the average person, playing sport that is less likely to result in injury could be a sensible consideration.

References

Fried R. The hyperventilation Syndrome Research and Clinical Treatment. The John Hopkins University Press. 1987. p41

Guthrie D, Moeller T and Guthrie R. Biofeedback and its application to the stabilization and control of diabetes mellitus. Am. J Clinical Biofeedback. 1983. 6:82-87

Tortora GJ, Anagnostakos NP. Principles of Anatomy and Physiology, Harper & Row, New York. 1984. pp412, 424

Youngsen R. The People's Medical Society. Blood Pressure: Questions You Have – Answers You Want. Thorsons. London. 1997. p28

Chapter 18

Epilepsy

People will happily discuss a broken leg, yet shy away from subjects like epilepsy. It is worthwhile to remember that epilepsy is a physical condition that has nothing at all to do with a person's intelligence or mental stability.

There are two main types of epileptic seizures - 'general' and 'partial', with five types of generalised seizures, and three types of partial seizures. For example, one of the 'generalised' types, the 'tonic-clonic' seizure (once known as 'grand mal') commonly involves muscle spasms and twitching, possible loss of consciousness, mental confusion and amnesia regarding the incident. On the other hand, also in the 'generalised' category, absence seizures (once known as 'petit mal') are hardly noticeable because the person may seem to be daydreaming. They might stop talking mid-sentence for a few seconds before carrying on where they left off. In the 'partial' category, 'complex partial' seizures 'usually start with a blank stare, followed by random activity. The person appears unaware of surrounding, may seem dazed and mumble. Unresponsive. Actions clumsy, not directed...' (Epilepsy New Zealand Fact Sheet 12).

Hyperventilation: A Cause of Epilepsy?

Epilepsy is not caused by anything structural in the brain. Instead it is a neurochemical problem and there are researchers all around the world who have linked hypocapnia and/or hyperventilation to epilepsy:

Gibbs et al (1940) reported:

> 'Considering all those links between carbon dioxide and epilepsy, namely that (1) the influence of carbon dioxide on the EEG, (2) the abnormal values of carbon dioxide in arterial and jugular blood of patients with petit mal and grand mal, and (3) the abnormal variation of carbon dioxide preceding grand mal seizures in such a way as to indicate a causal relationship, we may conclude that carbon dioxide plays a significant role in the aetiology of epileptic convulsions.'

Guyton, a well-respected scientist who has written numerous textbooks writes:

> 'In persons who are predisposed to epileptic fits, simply over breathing often results in an attack.'

Epilepsy: A Defence Against Hyperventilation?

It is well known that carbon dioxide has an enormous effect on the nervous system (Gardner 1989, Vansteenkiste 1991). Hyperventilation and the resulting hypocapnia and respiratory alkalosis stimulate nerves into action, dramatically reducing blood flow to the brain and inhibiting the release of oxygen to brain tissue (Guyton 1982). If this situation was forced to continue then the person would die, but it is not normally possible due to the person fainting when oxygen reaches a low pressure. When a seizure occurs, the brain becomes incredibly active, which produces a lot of carbon dioxide. For example, after thirty or forty-five seconds of convulsions, carbon dioxide pressure rises dramatically, to approximately the same point as it would if the person had held their breath (Magnaes 1974). This leads to the theory that a seizure is primarily due to low carbon dioxide and is a way of restoring normal levels.

Inhaling carbon dioxide is the most effective means of suppressing seizures and has virtually no known side effects say a number of researchers, who include Caspers and Speckmann (1972); Pollock (1949); Wang and Sonnenschein (1955); Woodburry and Kemp (1970). The only apparent drawback is the method of application. In theory then at least, by breathing correctly there is less likelihood of having seizures, and by learning the Buteyko Method control may be gained.

References

Caspers H. and Speckmann E.J. Cerebral pO_2, pCO_2 and pH: Changes during convulsive activity and their significance for spontaneous arrest of seizures. Epilepsia. 1972. 13. pp699-725

Epilepsy New Zealand Fact Sheet 12. Epilepsy: Recognition and First Aid. Based on information from the Epilepsy Foundation of America, 4351 Garden City Drive, Suite 406, Landover, MD, 20785.

Gardner WN, Bass C. Hyperventilation in clinical practice. British J Hospital Medicine. 1989. 41. pp73-81

Gibbs EL, Lennox WG, Gibbs FA. Variations in the carbon dioxide content in the blood in epilepsy. Arch. Neurol Psychiat. 1940. 43. pp223–239

Guyton. AC. Human Physiology and Mechanisms of Disease. W.B. Saunders Co. Philadelphia. 1982. p286

Magnaes B, Nornes H. Circulatory and respiratory changes in spontaneous epileptic seizures in man. European Neurology. 1974. 12. pp104-115

Pollock G.H. Central inhibitory effects of carbon dioxide. Journal of Neurophysiology. 1949. 12. pp315-324

Vansteenkiste J, Rochette F, Demedts M. Diagnostic tests of hyperventilation syndrome. European Respir J. 1991. 4. pp393-399

Wang R. I. And Sonnenschein RE. pH of cerebral cortex during induced convulsions. Journal of Neurophysiology. 1955. 18. pp130-137

Woodburry D. M. and Kemp J.W. Some possible mechanisms of action of antiepileptic drugs. Pharmacopsychiatry and Neuropharmacology. 1970. 3. pp210-226

Chapter 19

The Carbon Dioxide Syndrome

The Carbon Dioxide Syndrome is the result of a lifestyle that has too many stresses and insufficient physical exercise to maintain the level of carbon dioxide that is required to provide optimal performance.

The sayings 'Let nature take its course', and 'You will get over a cold in seven days if you take medication, and a week if you don't', are very often true because the body takes care of and heals itself providing it is given the necessary support. For example, within a few days of cutting your hand the skin has closed over and within two weeks you can barely see the wound.

External agents such as infection or wounding, a genetic mutation or poisoning, all contribute to ill health, but there are other conditions that are not caused by anything external. Arthritis is an example of the immune system attacking the body instead of a foreign object. Allergic asthma is another condition where the body reacts to harmless substances and in doing so, harms itself. A malfunctioning body may cause other conditions such as migraine headache, heart attacks, ulcers, high blood pressure and anorexia. When the body is so good at healing, why would it harm itself?

It is a basic Buteyko premise that continued stress will make the body malfunction but how it does this depends on your basic genetic make up. Chronic hyperventilation and the associated loss of carbon dioxide destabilises the whole body because carbon dioxide is the body's regulator. Any organ or body part that is damaged or inherently deficient could be badly affected when the body malfunctions.

Homoeostatic mechanisms keep the body functioning normally. For example, the core temperature will be essentially the same regardless of environmental temperature, providing exposure is not extreme. However, if stress on the body is excessive or long lasting, then the homoeostatic mechanisms may not be sufficient to keep the body functioning properly. Very often people do not acknowledge stress because it is such a customary part of life. For example, after driving for five hours the back, neck and shoulders are stiff but the person does not consider that they are stressed, rather that the muscles have cramped from sitting in the same position for such a long time. While this is true, it will be compounded by the fact that muscles constrict more efficiently when adrenaline flows, as it does when the person is stressed or exhilarated by driving at top speed.

Imagine that a person with a predisposition to heart disease constantly breathes more air than normal for a long period of time. This will cause:

- The heart to beat faster than normal
- Blood vessels to narrow and blood pressure to rise.
- Less oxygen and glucose received by tissue – including heart muscle.
- Potassium, calcium and magnesium excreted in greater quantities (the three minerals that have been shown to lower high blood pressure).
- Lipids (fats) in the bloodstream to rise and be deposited on the arterial walls.

These things mean that the person's heart will have to work harder and could lead to premature aging or damage.

Hans Selye (1984) states: "…. we are just beginning to see that many common diseases are largely due to errors in our adaptive response to stress, rather than to direct damage by germs, poisons, or life experience. In this sense many nervous and emotional disturbances, high blood pressure, gastric and duodenal ulcers, and certain kinds of sexual, allergic, cardiovascular, and renal derangements appear to be essentially *diseases of adaptation*."

Misdiagnosis of Syndrome

The symptoms of hyperventilation are many and varied and they mimic the symptoms of disease. For example, The Resistance Stage of the General Adaptation Syndrome allows a person to cope with prolonged stress while raising blood pressure and sugar levels above normal. But it can also provide doctors with incorrect data; for instance, if sugar levels are constantly high, it could be thought that the person has a problem with diabetes rather than suffering from prolonged stress and the associated hyperventilation.

In 1957, Dr. Lewis wrote about one hundred and fifty people with hyperventilation who had been previously misdiagnosed with at least one of the following conditions:

Acute rheumatic fever	'Allergic reaction'
Arthritis	Asthma
Brain tumour	Cardiospasm
Cerebrovascular accident	Cholecystitis
Cholelithiasis	Congenital heart disease
Cor pulmonale	Coronary heart disease

Emphysema	Epilepsy
Fibrosis	'Glands'
Hypertensive heart disease	Hyperthyroidism
Hyperventilation syndrome	Hypothyroidism
Insulin reaction	Islet cell tumours in pancreas
Myositis	'Nerves'
Peptic ulcer	Paroxysmal auricular tachycardia
Pheochromocytoma	Poliomyelitis
Respiratory tract infection	Rheumatic heart disease

When an illness is diagnosed, the person often starts drug treatment. Hyperventilating but otherwise healthy people taking medication for conditions that they do not have are bound to experience problems as the following examples show:

- The overuse of asthma reliever medications can contribute to worsening asthma (Crane 1989).
- People who overdose on corticosteroids or who take them for too long, find that their adrenal glands no longer make enough of the hormone to function properly. They need to continue taking the medication, often for the rest of their life (Cochrane 1987).
- Some medications, Clonidine Hydrochloride, Guanabenz Acetate, Mecamylamine Hydrochloride and Propranolol Hydrochloride for example, which are taken for high blood pressure, can have a rebound effect. This means that if they are stopped suddenly the blood pressure goes higher than it was prior to treatment (Govoni 1988).
- Decongestant medications such as Pseudoephedrine Hydrochloride, Naphazoline Hydrochloride, Oxymetazoline Hydrochloride, which are taken to combat sinus or hay fever problems also usually have a rebound effect, making the congestion worse than

previously noted (Govoni 1988).

- There are warnings regarding the overuse of antibiotics because bacteria become immune to them and the body becomes less effective at defending itself (Collingnon 1999).

Therefore the treatment of hyperventilation-related, rather than disease-related symptoms with medication is unlikely to be beneficial. And because hyperventilation goes untreated, then more symptoms may appear.

The Carbon Dioxide Syndrome goes Unrecognised

The people who are in the position to recognise the Carbon Dioxide Syndrome are doctors, yet this is not happening as frequently as it could (Magarian 1982). There are a number of possible reasons for this:

- Doctors are busy people who gain much of their knowledge from textbooks and medical journals.
- There is little monetary gain in researching chronic hyperventilation as it is not successfully treated with drugs and cannot be operated on. Therefore few articles are written about Buteyko in medical journals.
- Today chronic hyperventilation is not a common diagnosis as it was in the late 1800s and early 1900s (Baker 1934, Wood 1941).
- Dysfunctional breathing and its wide variety of symptoms is hard to recognise (Magarian 1982) and unlike blood pressure, heartbeat and sugar levels, breathing patterns are seldom checked, so it is possible to maintain an abnormal breathing pattern for years. It is almost certain

that Charles Darwin and Florence Nightingale suffered from dysfunctional breathing, but both were diagnosed with heart disease. Darwin in particular, had repeated illness and numerous symptoms of hyperventilation, yet lived to be seventy-three (Bowlby 1990) and Nightingale until she was ninety (Lum 1977).

Answers to Modern Day Health Problems

Buteyko has a basic premise that the cause of these modern day health issues (hyperventilation) is not being addressed, and therefore a cure is never realised. British chest physician L.C. Lum says that it is possible to breathe three times more air than the average healthy person without anyone noticing, and if no one notices the abnormality, then it will only become apparent when tests are done. It is commonplace to have blood pressure checked at each visit to the doctor but breathing is seldom checked apart from lung function tests, which are a check of the lungs rather than the breathing pattern. Breathing and blood gas pressures are probably only checked in a Critical Care hospital ward and while a person is ill, these are not expected to be normal. No one bothers to check them when a person is well, sitting on the sofa in their lounge room.

Drugs simply mask the symptoms and allow hyperventilation to continue rampantly, causing still more symptoms further down the track. In addition to this, the drugs themselves may create side effects, which then require extra treatment.

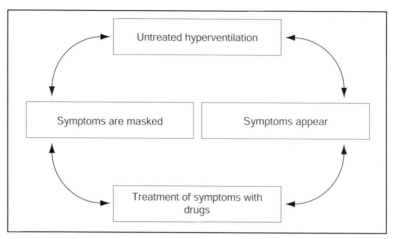

Figure 19:1. The Carbon Dioxide Syndrome goes unrecognized and untreated.

In addition to bad breathing habits, the other compounding problem of today is the lack of physical activity. When considering elderly people, it is obvious that the ones who remain active are the healthiest. Genetics must play a part in this, for example to avoid having a heart attack it is helpful to have a predisposition to a good vascular system. However, those who keep walking, playing bowls, gardening, or doing some other form of physical activity several times a week are more likely to live a long and healthy life than someone with the same genes who is a couch potato. This is also true for those who are not so old, and a healthier lifestyle can be started at any age.

In conclusion, regardless of whether deep breathing is a disease with multiple symptoms, or whether there are hundred of diseases that are exacerbated by low carbon dioxide tension, the solution is the same. Restoring normal breathing patterns undoubtedly helps hyperventilation-related health problems.

References

Baker DM. Sighing respiration as a symptom. Lancet 1934. 1. pp174-177

Bowlby, J. Charles Darwin: A New Biography. London: Hutchinson. 1990

Cochrane GM. Drug use in Respiratory Disease. Williams and Wilkins. Sydney. 1987. pp108-111

Collingnon PJ. Vancomycin-resistant enterococci and use of avoparcin in animal feed: is there a link? MJA. 1999. 171. pp144-146

Crane J, Pearce N, Flatt A et al. Prescribed Fenoterol and death from asthma in New Zealand, 1981-1983: a case control study. Lancet. 1989. 1. pp917-922

Govoni LE, Hayes JE. Drugs and Nursing Implications. Appleton and Lange. New Jersey. 1988

Lewis BI. Hyperventilation Syndrome: Clinical and physiological observations. Postgraduate Medicine. 1957. 53. pp259-271

Lum, LC. Breathing Exercises in the Treatment of Hyperventilation and Chronic Anxiety States. Chest, Heart & Stroke Journal. Spring 1977. 2. p1

Magarian GJ. Hyperventilation Syndromes: Infrequently Recognized Common Expressions of Anxiety and Stress. Medicine. Williams and Wilkins. 1982. 61. 4. pp219-236

Perera J. The Hazards of heavy breathing. New Scientist, 1988. Dec. pp46-48

Selye H. The Stress of Life, New York, McGraw-Hill. 1984. preface xvii

Wood P. Da Costa's syndrome (or effort syndrome). British Medical J 1941. 1. pp767–772, 805-811, 845-851

Chapter 20

Putting a Face to Buteyko

'What kinds of people want to improve their health naturally?' is a question that all Buteyko Practitioners ask themselves as they go about their business and is a little like asking 'How long is a piece of string?' The people who teach the Buteyko Method are also varied and this section of the book gives both clients and teachers a chance to explain why they have become so keen on the Buteyko Method.

Wanted: Opportunity to teach the Buteyko Method

Asthmatic with rejuvenated health wants to start up a Buteyko Practice in local area.

Creating good health by changing breathing patterns does not usually generate vast sums of money and often Buteyko Practitioners do not easily receive acceptance within their communities. Therefore it may seem a rather strange way of making a living to those with a conservative approach to life, yet surprisingly most of the people who teach Buteyko are fairly ordinary and not necessarily warrior types, or even serious about 'alternative' lifestyles. The vast majority are those who found the Buteyko Method life-changing and want to help others.

The People Who Teach Buteyko

Tess Graham was the first Buteyko practitioner to teach the Method in a medical trial outside of Russia. She was also the first Chief Executive Officer of the BIBH and tells us of her experience as a mother, physiotherapist and Buteyko Practitioner.

'As a physiotherapist, I worked in public and private hospitals and in private practice. I loved working with people with orthopaedic and sports injuries as usually I could help them get back to normal function. In respiratory wards 'success' wasn't always so easy. One role of the physiotherapist was to give breathing exercises to people with lung disorders in order to clear secretions from their lungs and maintain good air entry to all areas of the lungs. Now while this seemed like a good idea to help people with breathing problems, some patients found that a session of deep breathing (large, full breaths using the diaphragm) and coughing exercises could leave them exhausted and perhaps dizzy, albeit with less secretions in their lungs. However mucus could be back again when the next session was scheduled. Asthma was seen as an incurable and debilitating disease that medication management could relieve but the disease was seen as likely to be a lifelong affliction, needing lifelong medication.

I became interested in the Buteyko Method because my two eldest children each developed asthma at the age of three. Whilst maintaining them on the current best practice medical management, we tried all manner of complementary therapies. Some therapies reduced symptoms and medication needs temporarily, but the asthma progressed until the stage where my daughter was on a nebuliser one week in three and needing oral steroids occasionally and inhaled corticosteroids regularly. My son needed steroid medication seasonally.

When I read a health magazine article on the Buteyko Method, not only did Buteyko's theory make physiological sense, but it also made common sense! It explained so neatly why an asthmatic could bring on an attack by deepening their breathing, as they do by laughing, talking and exercising. It explained why deep-breathing exercises could bring on dizziness, coughing, and shortness of breath and fatigue. It explained why my eldest two children were more restless sleepers with sweaty heads and why I could stand at the doorway and hear them breathing in their beds at night, but could not hear my younger son. They were breathing more air than their younger brother! And when they breathed even more when excited, exercising or when they had an infection, they got asthma! Buteyko's theory explained all this and known physiology supported his theory. People with asthma are habitually over-breathing and it is a further deepening of breathing that can elicit the 'attack'.

I needed no further convincing. I took my children to learn the Buteyko breathing exercises. My daughter carried the nebuliser in its box in her backpack as we travelled to the course. The nebuliser never left the box again. Both my children were free immediately of the regular need for bronchodilators and were completely off preventers within six months. I could see the changes in their breathing. I could hear the changes. I observed other adults and children undergoing Buteyko training and saw similar dramatic positive results. That the practice based on Buteyko's theory works so well is further proof of the correctness of his theory.

I wanted no other mother to suffer the fear I had known and no other child to struggle to breathe as mine had. I underwent training to be a practitioner of the Buteyko Method in 1993. After completing my training I established the first Buteyko clinic in Canberra, Australia. I have since taught the Buteyko Method to over 3,500 people, and I also taught the Buteyko Method in the Brisbane clinical trial. At home I see my long-term study, my two former asthmatics are healthy and athletic. They have avoided spending the last ten years on bronchodilator and steroid medications and my younger son is an exceptional sportsman with remarkable endurance. He learnt as a five-year-old to run, and play sport with only nasal breathing.

I get great professional satisfaction from my clients achieving a quality of life that they feared was never to be theirs. As Professor Buteyko said, change will come from the bottom up. The people whose lives are improved by his method will bring about its eventual adoption as primary asthma management.'

Tom Fleming has the rare privilege of being the first person to teach the Buteyko Institute Method in an American hospital.

'While working at the Fairview Hospital in Great Barrington, Massachusetts, USA in 2000 I became involved in Buteyko when I was approached by an Emergency Room Doctor who asked me to read a study on Buteyko and see if I thought it had any value. Once I read it I could see that there was a great need for this method at the hospital because we were seeing a lot of asthmatics who were dependent on medication and not able to lead an active lifestyle.

We were able to receive training for people with mild asthma from a group in England and started our own Buteyko program. The hospital and local doctors were so supportive that I incorporated the Buteyko Method into my workday program, which helped many asthmatics. One was a nurse from the hospital who had asthma since she was 6 months old. After I taught her Buteyko, she has been able to go for one and a half years without any inhaler use, which had not been previously possible for over forty years.

Because we were getting such great results with our program with mild asthma, I wanted to do more and my hospital funded a month of training with BIBH trainer, Jennifer Stark in New Zealand. Since my expanded training I feel that I now have so much to offer the people of my community. I have completed a small study of the first 58 people that I have taught with these great results: Three weeks after class there was an 85% decrease in inhaler use as well as a 67% increase in quality of life. Twelve weeks later 62% were still having a quality of life growth. I also did a full year follow up and found that 100% had a quality of life growth and 85% had a continued decrease in inhaler use.

I now incorporate Buteyko in my Pulmonary Rehabilitation program at Fairview Hospital with people who have emphysema and have started to see that same relief look from these people as well, which gives me a great feeling. I believe that God sent Buteyko to me and I plan to work with it for as long as possible. I have a way to really help heal the suffering and fear that most asthmatics have of their condition.'

Mavis Riddel is a counsellor by profession who demonstrates that being under sixty is not a prerequisite to teaching Buteyko.

'It all started with a report by a well-respected journalist. You see I knew her delightful, down-to-earth family – we were neighbours for a brief time, when all our children were small. I knew they would have no truck with anything hocus-pocus, so when I read her newspaper article about how the Buteyko Breathing Method had benefited her son, I sat up and paid attention. I eagerly watched a subsequent presentation on the QED programme, of Sasha Stalmatski teaching the Method to some very severe, housebound asthmatics. I was astonished to see their progress – one person playing golf for the first time in years and another (housebound) able to go on holiday. Mind you, being a Scot, I was still a bit canny and it did seem a lot of money for a four-day (75 minutes a day) workshop.

I had asthma from the age of about four, probably inherited from my paternal grandmother and developed after a bad bout of whooping cough. I remember being a difficult patient – spoiled youngest child! I fiercely resisted the flour'n'mustard poultices, choked and gagged on tiny pills and became near hysterical at any mention of an injection. During one particularly bad attack, I had to inhale through a very large mask attached to a very large cylinder. In a second, my asthma symptoms had gone – and I was hooked on inhalers! Fortunately they got smaller. Over the years, I puffed my way through most of the "latest" medications, with varying results, ending up in my forties on the famous two, Ventolin and Becotide. There I would have stayed, on ever-increasing doses, had it not been for that article!

Of course, I went along to Sasha's workshop. After one week, I did not need Ventolin and after three months I took my last puff of Becotide. That was over five years ago. A year later, I trained as a practitioner with Russell Stark. At 65 years, I surely must have been the oldest Buteyko student practitioner ever! Since then, I have been teaching the Method very successfully in the southwest of England. Recently, I did an in-depth study of a group of asthmatics, youngest 5 years, oldest 79 years. The results showed that the Buteyko Breathing Method, practised properly, keeps asthmatics symptom free on minimal or no medication. My future goals? All children puffer free!'

Susan Neves was the first Buteyko Institute Practitioner in the USA.

'My first experience with asthma was when my daughter, then a toddler, had a severe attack which required hospitalization. The years that followed were punctuated with doctor and midnight emergency room visits. As she got older her attacks and their severity decreased and I breathed easier (literally!) but when I turned 35 I began to develop very severe hay fever. So severe, it was year round, and I was using a couple of large boxes of Kleenex a week. For years I got laryngitis so badly that every month or so I could not talk at all and had to take several days off from work each time to get my voice back. I went to an allergist and was prescribed shots, which I took (again for years). It helped, but every time we cut back, the symptoms would return. My skin became hypersensitive and very dry.

My second, third and fourth experiences with asthma came in rapid succession as three of my daughter's five sons developed asthma, two so severely that they were hospitalized on a regular basis, frequently in critical condition.

In early 1998 a friend of mine mentioned Buteyko when one of them was in hospital and suggested that it might help my grandsons. I was skeptical – it just seemed a little too unbelievable to me, but when I visited my grandson that night and watched him struggle to breathe, I decided to check into Buteyko. As I read about Buteyko on the Internet that night, I felt growing excitement because I knew it would work. It was beyond even my wildest expectations. The more I read, the more I knew I had to become a practitioner. I never again wanted to have to see my grandsons suffer the way they did. And I knew I wanted to help people like my grandsons lead normal and healthy lives.

209

I restructured my life and began my training six months later with Russell Stark. One thing that really surprised me was about a month after I took the course, my severe hay fever had receded, my extremely sensitive and dry skin had begun to 'normalize' and my perpetually dry mouth was perpetually moist. I was so surprised because I had never considered the idea that I suffered from chronic hyperventilation. My grandsons have not been in the hospital for asthma since they took the course and now lead normal lives. My hope is that every child suffering from asthma will have the same opportunity and experience they have had.

My life is very busy now as there are only a few Buteyko practitioners in the US, but we try to bring Buteyko to the awareness of the people who need it and to the medical community in a positive way. Several hundred people in the United States are walking around in better health because of learning Buteyko. I feel so grateful that life has given me the opportunity to help people in this way.'

Paul O'Connell was the second Chief Executive Officer of the BIBH and has been teaching Buteyko since 1994.

'I suffered from asthma for over twenty-five years having first been diagnosed with it at the age of five in the 1960s. I used a variety of drugs, yet the asthma continued to get worse, and I had two hospitalisations as a fifteen year old. From there it was a progression to nebulisers and oral steroids and still further deterioration. The asthma and medication severely restricted my lifestyle. This was particularly noticeable in my capacity to play sports where I lacked the ability and confidence to undertake many activities.

I tried many other health options as an adult, but these

only provided a small improvement in my asthma control. The Buteyko Method however, made a huge difference. I stopped needing asthma medications, and my symptoms kept getting less and less. I considered this a major breakthrough, not only for myself, but for other people that I heard about as well.

As a member of the public, my initial efforts at getting health authorities to look seriously at the Buteyko Method were unsuccessful, so I decided to train as a Buteyko Practitioner so I could help other people to get the great results I had already experienced. Teaching Buteyko is a wonderful experience as you consistently see people get significantly better in a very short space of time. Watching children transform over five days and knowing that they have changed the course of their health always makes me think I am privileged to have had the opportunity to become involved in Buteyko.

After unsuccessful approaches to health organisations in 1994, I helped to establish a professional organisation (the BIBH) to provide information on Buteyko for members of the public, the health professions and other health organisations. This has involved work in Australia, the United Kingdom and the United States. I intend to continue with this work so that as many people as possible will have the opportunity to benefit from learning the Buteyko Institute Method.'

Wendy Haddock was the first physiotherapist to teach Buteyko in England and played a major role in bringing Buteyko there.

'It was a happy accident that my husband was watching TV when "Frontline Scotland" came on with a 45-minute piece on Buteyko. Although I was very interested to see the results people were getting, the course seemed very expensive and wasn't validated by any authority that I was used to taking as a precedent, which made it hard for me not to be sceptical.

My mother's asthma was really bad and it was pure desperation that motivated us to further enquire and take the plunge on a course Alexander Stalmatski was running in Glasgow. She was terrified of the idea of taping up at night....so much so that I kicked my husband out of our bed and Mum and I taped up together. All I had was masking tape but even so once Mum had calmed down and got herself used to this seemingly bizarre idea she slept like a top and joy of joys, found herself not only alive the next day, but feeling so much better.

Watching Mum's life open up and her confidence grow as she mastered her condition was and is a delight. One year later we celebrated her recovery with a weekend in Paris. Watching her walk the feet off me, and whiz up and down the Metro gave that weekend a special joy, because before doing her Buteyko course she had been unable to get to Scotland to see us, let alone go to Paris.

Watching all this first hand inspired me to train as a practitioner. Partly as atonement for the many years I'd been going about my professional life encouraging people to deep breathe and cough but also to share with the many people like my Mum the liberation from the stranglehold of asthma.'

Bette Morris was the first nurse in USA to teach Buteyko.

'I have a daughter who had exercise induced asthma as a child and when the doctor treating her, barely able to breathe from asthma himself, prescribed an inhaler with praises about how they enabled him to exercise, I intuitively decided that was the last thing I would use for her. It obviously was not making him any better. We avoided the situations that gave her the breathing difficulty and got through it successfully. I was grateful that her problem was minor. But it left a lasting impression in my mind.

I am a registered nurse with more than thirty years' experience in the field of nursing. The kind of experience I had with my daughter as well as the way that I saw people treated (many conditions have painful and damaging conventional treatments) and the poor results they had with drugs, made me decide that there had to be a better way to help people and began a search for the other ways to help. I read an article by Dr. Paul Ameisen who had written a book about Buteyko and my immediate reaction was, "this is it".

I was very impressed by my first experience of Buteyko because I saw how much people improved in such a short time and it also cured my own problems of allergies and sinus congestion. I was also on the verge of sleep apnoea, but did not realize that until much later. I was also aware of the great difficulty I would encounter in teaching Buteyko in the US because there is much resistance from the drug companies and consequently the medical establishment to anything that does not involve drugs.

I continue to teach in spite of the resistance, because each time someone is helped to become more independent and in charge of their life, I feel a warm glow. I keep the faith that someday the drug empire will fall and then many more people will feel comfortable in trying this. Right now most people here are brainwashed into thinking that they cannot have control in their lives and drugs are the answer to everything. Buteyko has not become my sole source of income as I thought it might and I continue to do all the alternative therapies I have learned because each has its own place in health and people's beliefs.'

Tracey Steele is a Natural therapist in New Zealand who decided to add the Buteyko Method to her tools of trade.

'I was first introduced to Buteyko at the 1996 AGM of the South Pacific College of Natural Therapies in Auckland where I had qualified as a Naturopath, Medical Herbalist and Bowen Therapist. Buteyko's theory was impressive. He had looked beyond his medical training, quite outside the square and had created a method that ordinary people could learn to return to their original breathing pattern. I decided then and there that I wanted to teach it and use it myself.

It is now my preferred teaching method for my clients who benefit from every part of the Buteyko Method. In winter I recommend the Nose Clearing exercise almost daily. Anyone with insomnia, frequent night time urination, waking with mucus, snoring, or waking not refreshed, are asked to tape their mouth at night. All are delighted with the results. With the knowledge obtained from the Buteyko practitioner course and fully understanding hyperventilation, it has been hard to find an illness that Buteyko will NOT help.

In class and clinical situations where the technique has been taught, there has been satisfactory progress, reduction of symptoms and better quality of life in all cases. When the method is adhered to, the health benefits are phenomenal because Buteyko has amazing results. Fixing the cause of illness gets rid of symptoms and unnecessary medication.'

Sally Gething was the first Buteyko Practitioner in the North West of England.

'The Beginning: It was several years after I first heard of Buteyko before I took any active steps towards finding out anything about it because at that time, I had no particular interest in asthma. I did not have asthma or any breathing problems, nor to my knowledge had any of my friends or family. However I did know that asthma was an increasing problem in this country, with more children than ever before having the condition. However, a basic interest in the concept made me attend a seminar that was held near my home and within a few weeks I had started training to be a practitioner.

My Training: I began studying human physiology, the physiology of asthma and other breathing problems as well as the theoretical side of Buteyko. The practical side involved watching and assisting my trainer, Russell Stark to teach the Buteyko Method to asthmatics. Watching a week's course was startling because all the claims made in the Buteyko publicity came true right before my eyes. People who had been on up to 16 puffs of reliever on the first day, no longer needed any by the fifth day. This happened week after week and I saw over 50 people improve. As I learnt more about asthma, it was easy to see how people had ended up on so much medication, how debilitating it was, how sick people were, but most importantly, how in one week, they could be taught to change their breathing and start to leave asthma in their past.

My Business: Anyone considering being a Buteyko practitioner must realise that first and foremost they are running a business. Because Buteyko is a worldwide concern with practitioners, trainers and mentors often on the other side of the world, most of the time you work on your own promoting your practice, running courses in your area and trying do the job effectively. By following basic marketing principles I taught 100 people in my first year.

An Interesting Career: At first glance, it looks as if I

teach the same thing every week. In fact I do because I teach the Buteyko Institute Method. However because each person reacts to the exercises differently, has different problems, state of health, medical histories and is on different medication, by the second day of the course, I am tailoring the exercises for each person. By the fifth day, some participants have been able to make substantial changes to their breathing and consequently their condition, while others have made smaller changes. As a career, this makes for very interesting and varied work!

With Buteyko being worldwide, the initial discovery being made in Russia, work has an international feel to it and working in the United Kingdom is interesting because Buteyko is still in its initial stages. Educating people is the most challenging aspect of the job and I hope that in the future Buteyko will be used more widely as people learn that when they restore normal breathing patterns, their health improves.'

Peter Kolb has spent many years working with people who cannot get to a Buteyko course. He does this through a web site with email support. Peter also teaches small groups of people face to face.

'During my first year at medical school I developed some learning difficulties due to the stress of the huge volume of work. Since I spent all my time working and none of it exercising or relaxing, this work soon took its toll on me. My doctor decided that I needed a cocktail of Tofranil to help me forget the stresses, Valium to calm me down, and Dexadrine to pep me up again. The drugs worked a treat and I passed my first year well. But the following year I found I was unable to concentrate at all, and no amount of the drugs helped. My head was a ball of cotton wool. I could not assimilate a whole sentence because by the time I got to the end, I'd forgotten what the beginning was about. It was so serious I had to abandon my medical studies and later became a biomedical engineer.

I married and had children, one of whom turned out to be a severe asthmatic. We nearly lost him twice. We used to get up at two in the morning, shove a nebuliser full of chemicals down his little throat till he would shake uncontrollably and then repeat the performance two hours later. One of the hardest things for a parent to do is to stand by helplessly and watch your child deteriorate. What the doctors told us to do brought temporary relief, but there was no cure in sight for this dreadful disease. In fact, Alex was just getting worse. I would have done anything, paid any price to take this curse off my child.

My mother heard about this Russian breathing technique, which at the time didn't make any sense at all. But it had some good reviews and so I enrolled Alex. I wasn't very impressed by the first lesson and none of the others were either but when I picked Alex up the next day for the second lesson, he told me that he had used no bronchodilators at all that day. At first I didn't believe it, but when we walked into the lecture room that evening, the whole place resonated with a state of euphoria. Alex wasn't alone in having discovered that the Buteyko method works. Not only does it work but also dramatically and very rapidly. He never touched Ventolin again and a few months later he was weaned off his steroids. I converted his nebuliser into a solder sucker for my electronics work. We eventually had to trash all the expired medication and Alex became a strong and healthy young man.

I decided to use the education I worked so hard to get, viz my Masters in Medical Science, to try to understand how those dreadful allergic reactions were stopped by the Buteyko method. The bronchospasm bit made sense, but allergies? With just a little well-directed research I found that the Buteyko method reverses chronic hyperventilation (CHV). The physiological basis is very sound, simple, basic and astonishingly logical. Yet, as the writers of all the papers on CHV lament, very few doctors understand it or are even aware of it.

Not only did the hyperventilation theory explain why Alex had asthma, but it also explained the problems I had at university. Breathing too much is a very quick way to get sick. We have only some of the answers to good health, notably diet and exercise. But even Olympic athletes get asthma in spite of plenty of exercise and good diets. What many of them don't know about yet is that they need to avoid breathing too much to be healthy.

I still design and construct prototype electronic devices for health care for a living, but my mission has changed. I use just about all my spare time on disseminating and explaining Buteyko's theory. The sooner we can wean the millions of little kids right now hooked up to their nebulisers, the better.'

Dick Kuiper is a university lecturer and the first BIBH Practitioner in Holland.

'In 1994 I received a job offer from the Department of Agricultural and Horticultural Systems Management at Massey University, New Zealand, and before we fully realized what happened, my wife Judith, our children and I were on our way from Holland.

We spent six wonderful years in New Zealand, which is a beautiful country, but also one with the highest incidence of asthma in the world and as fate would have it, I developed asthma during our stay there. I had always taken breathing for granted, but now I know how frustrating and tiring it can be to have to struggle for every breath.

What appealed to me most about Buteyko is that it looks at the body as a whole, as a system, instead of fragmented parts, which really fits in with my idea of good science. I decided to do more research on the Buteyko method, and found a lot of material through the Internet: research papers, personal stories, newspaper articles. From what we read and heard from others a clear picture emerged: the Buteyko method has helped many people to gain control over their asthma and to reduce their medication. Except for a few doctors who are open-minded and willing to question the (blinding) beliefs of their own profession, it also is a method that is largely ignored by western medicine.

So I trained as a Buteyko practitioner and ran Buteyko courses in New Zealand for a time. At the beginning of 2000 Judith and I decided to move back to Holland, the pull of friends and family became too great. We started the Buteyko Instituut Nederland later that year, and since then I have been running group courses and giving individual training. We have our own web site now, and in July 2002 I teamed up with Dirk van Ginniken, another Buteyko practitioner.

Compared to New Zealand, working in Holland is, in some aspects, a little different. For example, we get fewer people with asthma and more people with chronic fatigue syndrome and stress induced chronic hyperventilation. Overall, people seem to be more stressed in Holland than I remember from New Zealand. It can be challenging at times, but I love what I am doing, the Buteyko method works and the method gets better known every day. Having worked in a university department where there was a keen interest in the diffusion of innovations throughout societies I know that it might take time before Buteyko's ideas will be accepted. As Schopenhauer, the great German philosopher, said around 1850: "Every truth goes through three stages: (1) first it is ridiculed; (2) then it is fiercely opposed; (3) and finally it is accepted as self evident." I expect Buteyko's theory to follow the same route.'

Debbie Meredith is an Australian pharmacist who has spent a great deal of time dispensing drugs. She also teaches Buteyko, helping people to improve their health with better breathing.

'Buteyko Breathing has certainly changed my life, both in regard to my health and my career. I first heard about Buteyko when my nephew Aaron Lumsdaine was teaching it in Perth. Aaron trained with Sasha Stalmatski and was a founding member of the BIBH. At the time, I didn't take much notice of it, until Aaron came to visit the family on the east coast. He told me about Buteyko and showed me some of his case histories. I was fairly skeptical, to say the least.

I had been a pharmacist for about 25 years, working in both hospital and community pharmacy. I have always been interested in natural health, and had studied a little about herbal medicine, reflexology and massage and had considered studying naturopathy years ago. I was very much aware of the adverse affects of medications, and concerned about their overuse. But I liked my job as Director of Pharmacy at Coffs Harbour Hospital and thought I would work there until I retired, many years hence.

Then Aaron told me that my breathing was terrible. "How else could I breathe?" I asked. "I've been breathing like this all my life. And besides, I'm perfectly healthy!" I thought I was fairly healthy, although I knew that I snored badly and I felt tired a lot of the time, which I thought was just from being middle-aged and working full-time and looking after a family.

Aaron invited me to attend a Buteyko course he was running while staying in my town, so I went along, curious but not really expecting much. How wrong I was! The theory of the Buteyko Method made sense and the physiology corresponded with what I had learnt many years ago in my university studies, but had never related to the practical aspects of breathing.

Within a few days of doing the Buteyko breathing exercises I had stopped snoring and had a lot more energy through the day. I realized that I had had sleep apnoea (my husband, Bruce, confirmed that I used to stop breathing often and start again noisily). I also saw the changes in the others in the course who had asthma, who ranged in age from a 4 year old to an 80 year old. Each evening they would all report "I haven't needed any relievers today." I was amazed, as I knew how dependent asthmatics normally are on their medications. I realized how effective the Buteyko Method is, and how many people could benefit from it.

Within a month my hay fever had disappeared (I had had it so long I thought it was normal, until it went away) and I had shed 5kg. I had also decided to train to teach the Buteyko Method.

Once I finished the training, I started running courses after work, while still working full-time. Then I took long service leave and ran daytime courses and travelled to other areas to teach the method. I returned to work at the end of my leave and resigned. Buteyko was to become my new career. I think most of the people who knew me thought I was crazy. I have never regretted that decision. I love being able to make a difference to people's lives, to teach them to take control of their health, and to see the dramatic changes in it. I work harder that I ever did in a job and financially I am much poorer, but this work is very satisfying. To hear people say "This has changed my life" is wonderful, and I hear it often. I will be eternally grateful to Aaron and to Professor Buteyko.

Stories From Those Who Learn Buteyko

To me, the Buteyko course meant a gateway to weight loss, improvement in overall fitness and lifestyle in general. I strongly recommend it to all who cling to their relievers like life preservers.' Daniel

People learn Buteyko for a variety of reasons. Most have got to the point where they are tired of using treatments that do not meet their expectations of being symptom-free or they are concerned about the possible side effects of their drugs. Others believe that prevention is better than cure and so enrol in a course before the condition or treatment becomes a real problem.

'I now have control of my asthma instead of my asthma having control of me.' Judy

'Buteyko is not dictatorial. It is about making informed choices about your condition in a supportive environment.' Esther

This section gives you stories written by a small sample of those who have chosen the Buteyko Institute Method to improve their health.

'Buteyko - the method, teaching and results are a dream come true. Every facet of life has improved. My Dad is a doctor and he says that physiologically he cannot fault it and adds that it is logical why it works.' Shelley

Lesley, 57 years old with severe asthma

'I developed asthma as a teenager after a bout of the flu but didn't have to take medication on a regular basis until I was in my early thirties. In my early forties I developed an infection after an operation, then had to have further surgery to clean up the infection. A couple of days after the second operation I couldn't move the peak flow meter but nothing further was done and I ended up with fluid on my lungs. While draining the fluid my lung was punctured and even after this repaired, my lung didn't immediately inflate. Following this my asthma really became severe.

I was fifty-seven when I heard about Buteyko and enrolled in a course. At that time I was taking:

*   250 mg Nuelin tablets twice a day. (The prescribed dose was 500 mg twice a day but I couldn't tolerate it)
*   One Volmax tablet before going to bed
*   2 - 3 puffs of Becloforte twice a day
*   2 puffs of Duovent 3 - 4 times a day
*   Nebulising twice a day with Ventolin

I was also having a course of 350 mg of Prednisone (70 x 5 mg) every 6 - 8 weeks. So I guess that I was correctly diagnosed as a chronic severe asthmatic. Apart from the constant asthma symptoms my feet constantly ached – when I woke in the morning the pain was terrible.

I did two Buteyko courses in 1997 and after doing this I went without any medication for three months but had to start back on the Becloforte after the flu. Looking back now, I think I was a bit hasty coming off the preventative medication. Four years later I attended another Buteyko course because three

223

months prior to it I caught a nasty viral infection that gave me a really bad cough. My doctor gave me 40 mg of Prednisone to help with that and I took 2 puffs of Becloforte twice a day until it settled. If I do some strenuous exercise or get a virus I take 1 - 2 puffs of Ventolin or Combivent.

Today I find the Buteyko exercises still help me with walking up steep slopes or stairs. My skin doesn't bruise or tear like it used to. Since my first course I have never had aching feet again! A few months after that first Buteyko course my doctor remarked that my eyes looked alive, they had lost that dull look I always had. She also said that my face had lost its bloated look and that she saw less of me than previously!

The hardest thing that I found about learning Buteyko was keeping my mouth shut and breathing through my nose! Plus slowing my breathing down when in a hurry or under stress. I still tape my mouth at night and do some Buteyko exercises when I watch television, do ironing, go out in the car or when I am sailing and walking. By doing this, my health is so much better than it was previously. I wish Buteyko had been available 25 years ago when I was first prescribed medication.'

Graeme, 50 years old with chronic asthma

'Recently I was at my doctor's for a renewal of my private pilot's licence medical. I asked him how long ago it was that I was prescribed my last Ventolin inhaler as all the ones that I had lying around had time-expired even though they were still reasonably full. I had forgotten when I did my Buteyko course so was astonished when he said 1998!!!

I have since found out that I did my course in November 1998, and I credit the lack of Ventolin to Buteyko. Before the course I was averaging 3 to 4 puffs of reliever per day. Now I don't have any reliever puffs at all! The only medication I take now is one puff of Flixotide at night, and I reckon I might even try dropping this soon.

The other day I went away on a bus trip for 8 hours and I didn't even bother to take along one of my time expired relievers. Normally I would have always had one in my pocket, but now I don't even worry about it.

One thing that I have noticed is my peak flow is not that great now that I don't use Ventolin. I blow about 350 to 360 on my peak flow meter, whereas before I did Buteyko I thought that I should be up in the 500's. However, there has been a slight improvement. The CAA [airline] medical people are puzzled why my last two lung function tests have shown an improvement when according to them they are expecting my asthma to worsen as I get older. Now they want me to provide daily peak flow tests for two weeks prior to my next medical, just to make sure that the last two medical results were not just because I was having a good day on the day that my medical was done!

What I have noticed is that I seem to need less air now, so that my lowered peak flow is not the problem that it was. Whenever I try a reliever inhaler, (which I have to do for my pilot's medical test because they take readings before and after using the medication), it hardly makes any difference to my peak flow, perhaps suggesting that I just have narrow airways. I keep telling the testing doctors, that I don't know why they keep getting hooked on peak flow. I tell them that I don't need that much air to fly with!!

When I was a baby, the Plunket [paediatric] Nurse told my Mum that I had a husky cry so I suppose I have always had something wrong with my breathing. I never heard about Buteyko until I was fifty. Since I had asthma for all my life it was difficult having confidence that Buteyko was going to work and I would say that it took two years for me to get the benefits that I have now.

As well as having virtually no asthma, I sleep a lot better. I am much more relaxed about my asthma now. It was always on my mind, especially if I was going away overseas. Now I don't even think about it. I walked the Abel Tasman track [one of New Zealand's great walks which takes an average four days] with a heavy pack and required no reliever. Five years ago I would have been gasping on an inhaler every one and a half hours to do anything like that. In fact I probably wouldn't have attempted it!'

Tim, 9 years old with mild asthma. His mother tells his story.

'Tim was first diagnosed as asthmatic when he was four years old with a persistent cough that kept him (and me) awake at night whenever he caught a cold. I gave him Ventolin but was concerned because it seemed to make him hyperactive. Over the next few years his asthma was a problem more frequently, and although he led a normal life he seemed to lack energy.

He only had one or two serious asthma attacks while growing into an older child but he never seemed really well either. If he ate ice cream or cheese he would start coughing and this could be quite dramatic. It was difficult to apply a diet. Then he developed sensitivity to cats, and would start wheezing if he visited anyone with a cat in the house. I was quite protective of Tim and stopped him going to school camps in case he had an asthma attack and made sure he came inside before the evening became too cold. I was concerned about him taking the steroid medication that the doctor wanted to prescribe so decided to try alternative health treatments.

Homoeopathic remedies seemed to make no difference, while osteopathic treatment helped considerably at first, but unfortunately it didn't last long. When I heard about Buteyko and was told the cost of the course it nearly put me off enrolling 9-year-old Tim, it seemed so expensive. But then I had already spent more than that on things that hadn't given him any lasting benefits. Also Buteyko had a 100% money-back guarantee that impressed me - no doctor or other health professional I had come across gave a similar guarantee.

Tim's improvement was obvious in the first couple of days of the course and his progress continued. His health that winter was so good I almost forgot that asthma had been a problem. He could get up early on frosty mornings and play hockey and even though we would take his puffer in case of emergencies, I no longer even thought about it.

Buteyko is not a 'quick-fix' cure, and you have to work at it. I think because asthma was never a big problem to him, and as Tim has grown into his early teens, he's not always conscientious about his breathing. His asthma can still be a problem if he comes down with a virus. But the amount of medication he needs is minimal - he doesn't need preventers and he might use 2-3 doses of Ventolin in total at these times. There have been two occasions when I took him to the doctor for an infection, but he has had no sign of asthma, to our doctor's amazement.

Another great benefit of the Buteyko course was how much I learned about asthma and the drugs prescribed for it. I now feel far more confident to help Tim with his condition, in both preventing him from having attacks and also in managing it if he does have problems. Our doctor supports our approach. I recommend any parents to enrol their asthmatic children. You won't regret it!'

Peter, 45 year old hay fever and sinusitis sufferer

'My son had done a Buteyko course which had helped him with his asthma so I decided to try it because I have had a problem with hay fever since I was a teenager. During spring and early summer, I had streaming, swollen eyes and a constantly blocked nose with sneezing fits that could last for minutes at a time. I tried many brands of antihistamine medication, but those that did help made me drowsy and I had to take time off from work. I was always breathing through my mouth because of my blocked nose.

Hay fever is not life threatening but it made me feel miserable. I had stopped going to places where there was long grass or flowering trees during the season. If I came into contact with something that triggered the hay fever, it would set it off for days and I felt that I was getting increasingly sensitive to pollens and scents. I had sinus congestion intermittently for the rest of the year.

I only enrolled in a Buteyko course out of desperation and started to learn the Method right in the height of the hay fever season. Because the inflammation process was already under way at that stage, I had quite a job to get the condition under control. I found that I could control the hay fever some of the time, but often at night my nose would block again. I found that with perseverance I made some improvement and I didn't have to resort to using medication.

I have incorporated the Buteyko way of breathing into my life so that I no longer habitually over-breathe; I am really conscious of keeping my mouth shut and breathing through my nose all the time, which no longer blocks. My sinusitis has virtually disappeared which has made my wife happier with lots fewer handkerchiefs to wash! My voice is less nasal. The best thing though, is that I can sleep far better - having a good night's sleep is wonderful. I sleep the whole night, don't snore (my wife loves that bit), and don't wake in the morning with a dry, sore throat.

Buteyko wasn't easy for me at first, but the long-term results have proved really useful. I sometimes still have a bit of trouble with the hay fever season, but I now feel better equipped to help myself through it, and I'm more confident about applying the Buteyko techniques before it becomes too bad. Knowing what to do before the hay fever starts is a great help. Even during the rest of the year Buteyko has made a significant difference to my health - I don't seem to catch as many colds as I used to and my sense of smell has improved.'

Janna, 39 years old with M.E./C.F.S.

Janna is a single mother and in the summer of 1995, six months after her daughter was born she had to stay in bed for three weeks, totally exhausted. Even after this she could hardly lift her arms and felt chronically tired, with periods of complete exhaustion. In the mornings she would often make a list of things to do for that day, but then found she only had the energy to do one of them, and even that task was often not completed, so life became very frustrating.

'Every day I was juggling with the energy I had, I often was uncertain of how to manage till the end of the day. I used to be energetic and fit, spending my holidays in the mountains and walking with 15 kilos on my back. But because of my fatigue I thought that this was over for good. I was young, but felt old.'

229

She also suffered from hay fever and eczema but always feeling weak and tired was the worst part of her illness. 'My muscles always felt tired, and when I tried to do something physical I had to pay for it later. I once helped my father for half an hour in the garden. Afterwards I was completely exhausted and it took me days to recover.'

But this is all behind her now, since attending a Buteyko course she has much more energy and her constant fatigue is gone. 'I went to an information evening on the Buteyko method and decided to try it. I also started to observe my breathing and noticed that I was breathing through my mouth a lot, quickly out of breath, and sighing a lot. I was just breathing much too much. When I entered the course my Control Pause was 6 seconds. By the end of the first week I had built it up to 20 seconds. Soon I noticed I was becoming less tired, but only when I went away for a weekend to visit a friend, did I realise how well I was actually doing. It was a long trip to see her and the rest of the day we were going out, we talked all night, and went to bed late. Amazingly I felt fine the next day!'

She has noticed other differences as well, such as not getting sick as often, she feels more calm and relaxed, and she is not as sensitive to sugar any more. 'I can now eat a piece of cake again when there is a birthday party, and I really wouldn't have tried that when I was still chronically fatigued. I also have noticed that I don't become weak and dizzy when I get hungry and I don't have to eat straight away like I had to.'

Her hay fever has also reduced but the big difference for her is without a doubt that she has regained her energy. 'Of course I am sometimes tired at the end of the day, just like everybody else. But I don't struggle through the day any more. I have much more energy, I bike with my daughter, I bought a dog who needs a lot of attention and I notice that I am not out of breath as quickly.'

Jenny, 30 year old panic attack sufferer

'I have young children, and life is pretty full without having the worry of panic attacks and claustrophobia. For over 15 years I had trouble sometimes with bouts of feeling very uncomfortable and fearful in places such as supermarkets, banks or waiting in queues.

On bad occasions I would feel tingling in my arms and my hands would turn cold. My heart raced and my breathing would go out of control. I would feel as if I was going to faint, although this only happened to me once. I believed it was something I had to learn to handle myself, but I really struggled to overcome it. Most of the time I kept on doing things but a couple of times I didn't go out to dinner at a restaurant because I didn't think I would be able to cope with the 'closed in' feeling. There were periods when the attacks were particularly bad. I think that this was connected to stress at work, when lots of demands were placed on me.

I didn't discuss the panic attacks with my doctor as I was afraid that I would be given something like Valium. I have read of people who were suffering from panic attacks being told they had psychiatric disorders - that really scared me. I had no idea it was so common, or that it would be helped so easily by breathing retraining.

In 1996 I had a dentist's appointment, and had my worst panic attack while in his waiting room. I passed out, and after that decided that I had to get help to overcome the problem. A friend told me about the Buteyko Method and I enrolled in the course.

It is so much easier when you understand the physiology of over-breathing. When you can see what is happening in a panic attack, half the battle is won. By practising the exercises, it meant that I could go to all the places that previously made me feel claustrophobic, without any problems. Any attack I now have is on a much reduced scale. I can control them - I am very aware of what causes them and I have this wonderful feeling of empowerment. I control the feeling - and know that I can overcome it. My doctor has received information about this technique and is very supportive of my using it. I like to tell people about Buteyko so they can be helped as I was.'

Sandra, 43 year old with bronchiectasis and asthma

'Three years ago I was desperate to find a way of relieving my quite serious asthma and bronchiectasis. I also wanted to cut down on the large amounts of steroid medication that had seemed necessary for years to keep me stable. I was looking for anything that would make some difference so I had tried various alternative health remedies, but none really helped me. I had no energy - even hanging out the washing was exhausting and lifting up my arms to do my hair was an effort. I was worn out just walking up steps, and life itself seemed like hard work. I also had trouble sleeping at night, and was unable to relax because my heart was always racing. I was constantly thirsty, and my arms were often numb.

After seeing a newspaper advertisement, I attended a Buteyko course and learned the control techniques that have changed my whole approach to living. Within a week of learning the Buteyko method, my energy levels increased and I just felt so much better. I followed the programme conscientiously and soon found that my symptoms were disappearing.

I could do the daily chores easily, and friends and family started to comment on how my health had changed for the better. I can do it all now - vacuuming, gardening, walking – just a normal part of daily life without having aching muscles. My hay fever has greatly improved and I feel so much more positive.

Pretty soon after the course I was able to cut down on all my medication and I now control my condition with the minimum amount, with my specialist's approval. It seems hard to believe that something so simple could make such a difference to me. Once the theory behind Buteyko was explained to me, it really made sense. I keep doing the exercises because they work.'

I have been weaned off of all the other medications under my doctor's supervision. Buteyko is a Godsend! Too often, doctors over medicate without having a full picture of what is actually going on. When that fails, they make you think that it's all in your head. Buteyko was the answer to my prayers and I will be eternally grateful that I happened upon your web site.'

Donna, has found using the Buteyko On Line Home Education Kit enormously helpful in learning the Buteyko Method.

'I was always a mouth breather and a chest breather as well, but my asthma symptoms only appeared 6 years ago. As time went on they got a little worse but I always felt that I could deal with them. The inhalers never seemed to really help.

I take very good care of myself. I don't drink or smoke, I watch what I eat and I exercise five times a week. Last year my husband and I were on vacation when I had a bad asthma attack. It scared me terribly. I literally thought I was going to die.

When I got back home I went to my doctor. He agreed that I was in a lot of distress and made me use a nebuliser in the office. He put me on steroids, which I took for 7 days. I was put on Singular, Advair and Proventil. Even after being on all this medication I still didn't feel 100%. That's when I decided this was crazy and I started doing my own research on the Internet. I came across the Buteyko New Zealand web site. There are few Buteyko classes in the USA and none close to where I live so I had no choice but to order the Home Kit.

Triggers for me are as follows: stress, changes in barometric pressure, the smell of strong perfumes and cleaning agents, and certain foods such as strawberries. The triggers still exist today but for the most part I am able to keep things under control when I am exposed to them. I can't do anything about barometric pressure or certain stressful times in my life. However I am more aware now, and the Kit literally taught me to breathe properly. Buteyko helps me to at least feel as though I have some control in the matter.

At the time of writing, I have only had to use my inhaler to deal with one attack in the past six months. And, since I know how to breathe properly now, the inhaler actually did its job. I used the inhaler twice that day and did my breathing exercises. What would have turned into a two-week episode in the past was over in just the one day.

Tom, also tells his story with teaching himself the Buteyko Method:

'I've been practising and refining my understanding of the Buteyko Method for approximately 3 years now without access to a teacher, relying solely on video and printed materials about the Buteyko Method. Over time I have adjusted my diet and lifestyle to help reduce the nagging persistence of nearly 23 years of adult onset asthma that varied from mild to severe, depending on the time of year here in Las Vegas, Nevada. The modifications in diet and lifestyle helped to reduce, but not entirely eliminate, my asthma condition. This year was different, however, and I believe I have the Buteyko Method to thank for this.

I did not have to resort to drugs during our spring allergy season which, I understand, has been one of worst in recent memory for Las Vegas. For me, this was nothing short of miraculous. I do the Buteyko exercises in the evening during the work week, and mornings and late afternoons on weekends.

I recently helped my daughter and son-in-law move out of one upstairs apartment and into another. By pacing myself and regulating my respiration rate with the Buteyko Method, I experienced no breathing difficulties whatsoever. At times, I could feel my body wanting to increase its respiration rate more than was really necessary for the level of exertion I was experiencing as I carried box after box upstairs. But I resisted and instead, took short, shallow breaths.

It was approximately a year ago that I threw out my asthma prescription medicines. By that time they had expired and I made no effort to renew the prescriptions. I did use a herbal tincture last year—which was very effective when I did get into respiratory distress, but only a few times. This year—and for the first time in many, many years, I did not need to resort to medicines of any kind for asthma or allergies. Without question, the Buteyko method is the crown jewel in my personal program of asthma control and allergy prevention. Dr. Buteyko deserves the Nobel Prize in Medicine for his life-saving research into the cause and cure of respiratory distress/failure and related medical ailments!'

Chapter 21

Learning the Buteyko Method

There are a variety of ways that you can learn the Buteyko Method and attending classes and teaching yourself are discussed in this book.

The best way to learn how to use the Buteyko Method is by attending classes with a well-trained Buteyko practitioner and today there are Buteyko classes held in most countries. To find out where your nearest practitioner is, check in your telephone book, look for the practitioner guide at: *www.buteyko.co.nz* or email: *courses@buteyko.co.nz* detailing your country, province or state and nearest city.

Attending Classes

The Buteyko Institute Method programme consists of five ninety minute sessions spread over one - two weeks with as many follow up sessions as are required. Each day new information is learned, and this builds to produce substantial education about breathing and hyperventilation-related conditions. Course attendees learn how to take part in everyday activities such as eating, talking and exercising without hyperventilating.

At the same time the Buteyko exercises are changing each person's automatic breathing pattern, so that overall, breathing becomes more normal and less attention is required to breathe correctly while doing these everyday activities.

The programme is tailored to suit each participant and strategies are developed to assist in the alteration of breathing patterns for any specific problems. Any reduction of drugs is done with the assistance of the participant's medical practitioner, ensuring that all progress is done safely and carefully.

Teach Yourself

While not the perfect way to learn Buteyko, some people who cannot get to a course teach themselves to use the Buteyko Method. The most common ways of doing this are:

- Using The Buteyko Asthma Management Home Education Kit (visit: *www.buteyko.co.nz/products/* for further details - produced by the authors of this book).
- Accessing Peter Kolb's self-help web site: (*www.wt.com.au/~pkolb/buteyko.htm*).
- Reading books about Buteyko.

It can be difficult to teach yourself something physical just by reading about it, so self-help books are possibly the most difficult way of doing this.

With Peter's site you will get ample feedback and support from other people who are already using the Method. They will give you ideas on how to tackle the problem of learning on your own.

Knowing how hard it is to learn something without seeing it, we developed our Home Education Kit with a video, along with an instruction manual, workbook and email support to make the Method easier to learn. Getting to a practitioner however, is the best way of all.

Learning to Teach Buteyko

Like learning to use the Buteyko Method for your own health, there are a variety of ways to learn to teach the Method. The approach that we recommend is authorised by the Buteyko Institute of Breathing and Health. It is a comprehensive course that has three distinct sections and takes approximately nine months to fully complete, but you can be teaching sooner than this.

The first section of the training is to read selected books about Buteyko, hyperventilation and related topics and to complete some assignments on these topics and the proposed Buteyko business.

The second section takes at least four weeks to complete and is a 'hands on' or practical component. During this time the trainee takes part in a number of Buteyko courses by assisting, co-teaching and teaching solo while being observed by the trainer. At the same time the person attends several hours of theory and discussion on the Method, drug therapies, conditions Buteyko is used to treat and other relevant topics.

The third section of the training is teaching clients without observation by the trainer and providing case histories on these people to the trainer. In addition to these case histories assessment is done by two written examinations, the ability to teach in front of the trainer and a number of oral tests.

To find out more about becoming a Buteyko Practitioner email for further information to *training@buteyko.co.nz*

The Future of Buteyko

To date there has only been one trial published on the Buteyko Institute Method and this was on using it to treat asthma. So far there have been no trials on any other condition. The results of this trial showed a 96% reduction in reliever medication, a 49% reduction in preventer medication and a 71% reduction in symptoms. Other trials on asthma have been undertaken with similar results but they have yet to be published. Anecdotally these results are reported in Buteyko classes every week. In spite of these impressive results, Buteyko is still not generally accepted by mainstream medicine. This comes as no surprise when you consider that it took thirty years for doctors to learn to wash their hands and also the number of trials promoting the value of drugs published every year.

In spite of this lack of acceptance, the number of people learning Buteyko and teaching it is growing at an enormous rate. In 1996 the Buteyko Method was taught in only two countries outside of the USSR and seven years later it is taught in more than twenty. It has made these inroads due to personal and financial sacrifices from people who have benefited in some way from the Buteyko Method. Lack of finances and public awareness of the Method is hampering its potential growth, yet due to its extreme effectiveness, it is still growing at this remarkable pace.

Members of the Buteyko Institute of Breathing and Health expect the Buteyko Method to become accepted into mainstream medicine, and hopefully this will come sooner, rather than later. As the medical profession gains more understanding of chronic hyperventilation and the realisation that drug therapies are not the sole answer, and often cause more problems than the original health issue, it will look outside of the current medical model for answers. Buteyko not only explains why diseases of modern life are growing at an alarming rate, but it also provides an easy solution with no negative side effects.

It would be nice to think that in ten years' time when a child is diagnosed with asthma, they are taught to normalise their breathing pattern instead of being put on a lifetime regime of potentially dangerous drugs. You can help this to happen by bringing the awareness of Buteyko to members of your community, and especially to your doctor. In reality, there needs to be more clinical trials on the Buteyko Method, and your doctor has a better chance of getting this to happen than possibly any other person.

Glossary

Acetylcholine - neurotransmitter that stimulates skeletal muscle contraction.

ACTH – adrenocorticotropic hormone that is produced by the pituitary gland and stimulates the adrenal cortex..

Addison's Disease – disorder caused by an undersupply of glucocorticosteroids. The main symptoms are weak muscles, weight loss, low blood pressure, dehydration and lethargy.

Adenoids – pharyngeal tonsils.

Adrenal cortex – the outer portion of each adrenal gland that secretes various hormones.

Adrenal medulla – inner portion of each adrenal gland that secretes adrenaline and noradrenaline.

Adrenaline – a hormone that stimulates the sympathetic nervous system via the adrenergic nerve receptors. It increases blood pressure, heartbeat, glucose release and opens up the airways.

Adrenergic nerve receptors – nerve receptors that either respond to or release adrenaline.

Allergen – an antigen that provokes an allergic reaction.

Allergy – an extra-sensitive reaction that occurs after exposure to a particular allergen.

Alveoli – air sacs in the lungs where gas exchange occurs.

Alveolus - one air sac

Anaemia – a condition where the number of red blood cells is lower than normal.

Angina - pain in the chest that is related to reduced blood circulation in the heart.

Antibody – a substance produced by the body to neutralise, inhibit or destroy an antigen.

Antigen – a substance that is introduced into the body and either reacts with antibodies or causes them to be formed.

Antihistamine – a medication that neutralises the action of histamines.

Antioxidant – a substance that prevents or delays the deterioration caused by oxygen.

Asthma – a condition where periodically the airways narrow, swell and become clogged with mucus making it difficult to breathe. In between these periods, breathing is unaffected.

Atherosclerosis – a process where fatty substances such as cholesterol or triglycerides are deposited in the arterial walls. This damages the walls, which react by absorbing more cholesterol and increasing the size of smooth muscle found within the walls, narrowing the arteries.

Autoimmune disease – a disease where the body attacks its own tissues.

BIBH – Buteyko Institute of Breathing and Health Inc. An association formed for and by Buteyko Practitioners in Australia, but which today has worldwide membership.

Bicarbonate ion (HCO_3) – an important regulator of blood pH.

BIM – Buteyko Institute Method. The way the Buteyko Method is taught and supported by BIBH members.

Blood gases – normally refers to the pressure of oxygen and carbon dioxide in the bloodstream, but may also refer to other gases that are found there, such as nitrogen.

Bronchi – plural of bronchus, which is a large airway.

Bronchiectasis – a condition where the airways become

chronically dilated and corrugated.

Bronchitis – a condition where the airways are inflamed.

Bronchodilator – medication that opens airways either by relaxing smooth muscle contraction or by preventing the contraction.

Carbon dioxide - a gas that is both produced and required by every living cell. Primarily used in regulation of many bodily functions.

Carbonic acid (H_2CO_3) - an important regulator of the blood pH.

Cardiac neurosis – neurocirculatory asthenia or hyperventilation syndrome.

Corticosteroid – a steroid manufactured by the adrenal cortex and also synthesised for use as a medication. It is believed to suppress inflammation, the immune response and ACTH production.

Cerebrovascular accident – destruction of brain tissue caused by a problem with the blood vessels that supply the brain. Commonly called a stroke.

Cholecystitis – inflammation of the gall bladder.

Cholelithiasis – a condition where the person has gallstones.

Chronic Fatigue Syndrome – a state of increased, excessive and prolonged fatigue, with general malaise and a loss of capacity to respond to stimulation.

Cilia – tiny hair-like structures that move rhythmically to move either the cell they are attached to or a mucus blanket.

Comatose – the state of coma or profound unconsciousness.

Congenital heart disease – heart disease that was present at birth.

Congestive heart disease – a state where the heart is incapable of supplying sufficient oxygen to the body.

Controller – long-acting reliever medication used in the treatment of asthma.

Cor pulmonale – diseased lungs or diseased blood vessels that are found within the lungs causing a heart condition.

Coronary heart disease or Coronary artery disease – a disease of the arteries within the heart, which results in heart muscle receiving inadequate supplies of oxygen. It is compounded by atherosclerosis and spasm of the arteries.

Corticosteroid – one of the steroids manufactured by the adrenal cortex, of which there are two major groups – glucocorticoid and mineralocorticoid. They are also synthesised and used clinically to treat asthma, arthritis etc. because one function of glucocorticoids is to inhibit the immune response.

Cushing's syndrome – a disorder caused by oversupply of glucocorticosteroids. The main symptoms are thin arms and legs with a plump body and face, flushed facial skin and poor wound healing.

Cystic fibrosis – an inherited disease that affects the lungs, pancreas, salivary and sweat glands.

Deep vein thrombosis (DVT) – a blood clot that occurs in a deep vein, such as found in the leg.

Diaphragm – large, dome-shaped muscle that separates the lungs from the stomach area. It is the muscle used primarily for breathing.

Dysfunctional breathing – an abnormal breathing pattern that has been shown to cause a number of symptoms, such as breathlessness, chest tightness, chest pain, light-headedness, tingling, numbness and anxiety.

Emphysema – condition where the alveoli are enlarged and damaged.

FEV_1 – Forced Expiratory Volume – how much air it is

possible to exhale in one second.

Extracellular fluid – blood and other fluids found outside of tissue cells.

Fibrosis – an abnormal formation of fibrous tissue.

Floppy airways - condition where a small trigger causes the airways to narrow or collapse.

Free radicals - excess oxygen molecules in the tissues that cause oxidative destruction within the cells, damaging the cell's metabolic systems.

Gastric reflux – reverse flow of the stomach contents into the oesophagus.

General Adaptation Syndrome – the wide range of bodily events that occur to deal with stress, so named by Canadian Doctor Hans Selye.

Glucocorticosteroid – one of the corticosteroids that are manufactured by the adrenal glands. They are primarily involved in metabolism of carbohydrates, fats and proteins, inhibition of inflammatory and allergic responses and growth of connective tissue. Also synthesised and used in the treatment of asthma, arthritis etc.

Glucose ($C_6H_{12}O_6$) – a sugar that is the major source of energy for every cell in the body.

Glycogen - a compact store of glucose in the liver and muscles

Haemoglobin - a protein found in red blood cells that carries oxygen.

Histamine – a substance that is released when cells are injured to prevent further damage to the body. It causes inflammation, widened and leaky blood vessels, lower blood pressure, smooth muscle spasm, increased heartbeat, mucus and gastric acid production.

Homoeostasis – the tendency towards maintaining a normal environment within the body.

Hydrogen ion (H^+) – a chemical element that is used to identify the pH of a substance.

Hypercapnia – an abnormal excess of carbon dioxide in the bloodstream.

Hypertension – blood pressure that is abnormally high.

Hypertensive heart disease – damage to the heart caused by high blood pressure. The heart uses more energy to pump blood when blood pressure is high and this results in an enlarged heart, which consequently requires more oxygen to function.

Hyperthyroidism – an overactive thyroid gland. The main characteristics are an enlarged thyroid, high metabolic rate with weight loss and lots of energy, protruding eyes, rapid pulse, flushed and moist skin.

Hyperventilation syndrome (H.V.S.) – a state where hyperventilation is maintained over a lengthy period and results in a wide variety of symptoms in many different parts of the body. The main characteristics are breathlessness, dizziness, fatigue, chest pain and rapid or pounding heartbeat.

Hypotension – abnormally low blood pressure, especially a sudden drop in pressure.

Hypothyroidism – an underactive thyroid gland. The main characteristics are a roundish, puffy face, slow heartbeat, lethargy, muscular weakness and a tendency to gain weight easily.

Hyperventilation – breathing more air than is required for metabolism.

Hypocapnia – abnormally low pressure of carbon dioxide in arterial blood. It is always caused by hyperventilation.

Hypoventilation – breathing less air than is required to meet the demands of metabolism.

IgE – Immunoglobulin E – an antibody that is formed in response to antigens entering the body.

Insulin – a hormone produced by the pancreas that decreases blood glucose levels.

Keto acid – an acid that is a precursor of amino acids. E.g. Pyruvic acid is a keto acid and is the precursor of the amino acid alanine.

Ketone – substance such as acetone or acetoacetic acid, which is formed primarily by the rapid breakdown of fats.

Lactic acid – an acid that is formed by the anaerobic metabolism of carbohydrates.

M.E./C.F.S. – Myalgic Encephalitis / Chronic Fatigue Syndrome. A state where the person experiences excessive and chronic fatigue along with any number of other symptoms such as painful joints, headaches.

Metabolic acidosis – blood pH less than 7.35, which is not caused by an excess of carbon dioxide, but instead usually by an abnormal increase in metabolic acids such as lactic acid, or by the loss of excessive bicarbonate ions which can occur with diarrhoea.

Metabolic alkalosis – blood pH that is greater than 7.45 and is not caused by a loss of carbon dioxide, but instead usually by taking too many alkaline drugs or by excessive vomiting of the stomach contents and loss of hydrochloric acid.

Metabolism – the number of kilojoules it takes to stay alive and to function or the sum of all the chemical processes and physical reactions in the body.

Minute Volume – amount of air breathed over a one-minute period.

Myositis – inflammation of skeletal muscle.

Neurasthenia – a condition with chronic weakness and fatigue.

Neurotransmitter – a substance that either excites or inhibits the target cell.

Nitrogen – gas that forms approximately 78% of the

atmosphere.

Oxygen – gas that is essential for all life and assists in supplying energy to the body by combining with glucose.

Parasympathetic nervous system- one of the two parts of the autonomic nervous system that causes activities which both restore and conserve energy.

Paroxysmal auricular tachycardia – heartbeat that alternately becomes rapid and then slows.

Peptic ulcer – an ulcer that is found within the part of the gastrointestinal tract that is exposed to hydrochloric acid.

Peripheral circulation – blood vessels on the surface or outer parts of the body.

pH – 'potential hydrogen'. The measure of acidity or alkalinity of a substance. The pH scale extends from 0 to 14, with 7 being neutral. Values lower than 7 are increasingly acidic and those higher 7 are increasingly alkaline.

Pheochromocytoma – a tumour in the adrenal medulla that causes hypertension and an increased secretion of adrenaline.

Poliomyelitis – an acute viral disease that may cause muscle atrophy and paralysis.

Polyp – a growth on a stem that protrudes from a mucous membrane.

Preventers – medication used in the treatment of asthma to prevent asthma symptoms and the need for reliever medications.

Pulmonary – pertaining to the lungs.

Pyruvic acid – a break down of glycogen. When pyruvic acid combines with oxygen, it produces carbon dioxide, water and a large release of energy.

Raynaud's Disease – a condition where peripheral circulation is so poor and so greatly affected by the release of adrenaline that lack of blood flow causes damage to the skin, especially that of the hands, feet, lips, nose and ears.

Relievers – short-acting medication used in the treatment of asthma to relax smooth muscle and open up narrowed airways.

Respiratory Acidosis – a state where the blood pH is less than 7.35 and is caused by abnormal breathing patterns that create an excessive retention of carbon dioxide.

Respiratory Alkalosis – a state where the blood pH is greater than 7.45 and is caused by hyperventilation that creates an excessive loss of carbon dioxide.

Respiratory centre – nerves in the brain stem that regulate breathing.

Rhinitis – hay fever, inflammation of the nasal passages that is usually characterised by excessive mucus production in the nose.

Schizophrenia – a severe psychiatric disorder that can be characterised by withdrawal from reality, hallucinations, delusions or bizarre behaviour.

Sinus – a hollow place in the body, such as found in the nose.

Sinusitis – commonly known as inflammation (and often infection) of the nasal sinus.

Skeletal muscle - muscles attached to tendons and bones that can usually be contracted and relaxed with conscious thought.

Sleep apnoea – a condition where there are many brief attacks of ceasing to breathe automatically.

Smooth muscle - involuntary muscle that is found wrapped around all hollow parts of the body. It cannot be contracted or relaxed with conscious thought, but responds to chemical stimuli, such as carbon dioxide pressure and histamine.

'Steroids' – glucocorticosteroids that are synthesized and used in the preventive treatment of asthma.

Stress – The bodily changes that are activated by the General Adaptation Syndrome when the person is exposed to any stimulus such as physical injury, worry, infection etc.

Stressor – something that causes stress.

Sympathetic nervous system – one of the two parts of the autonomic nervous system that primarily causes activities that stimulate the body.

TMJ (Temporo-mandibular joint) - part of the cheekbone where the lower jaw connects to the skull.

Tonsil - small mass of lymphoid tissue, commonly referring to those found on either side of the pharynx.

Ventricle – a chamber of the heart and also a section of the brain.

Work of breathing - the amount of energy it takes to breathe.

Index

Heart attack 184, 195, 201
Heartbeat 11, 15, 30, 43, 44, 69, 150, 152, 153, 155, 199
Henderson, Yandell 19, 161, 176
Hidden Hyperventilation 45, 74, 79, 132, 158, 178, 180, 183, 189
High blood pressure 48, 69, 181, 184, 195, 196, 197, 198
Homeostasis 11, 15, 52
Homeostatic mechanism 15, 196
Hormone 19, 67, 133, 159, 183, 187, 198
Horse Rider 79
Hydrogen ion 21, 189
Hypertension 9, 67, 122, 181, 183, 185
Hyperthyroidism 73, 198
Hyperventilation 39, 40, 41, 42, 43, 47, 50, 51, 55, 74, 88, 95,
146, 149, 150, 151, 153, 155, 179, 183, 192, 193, 198
Hyperventilation - Asthma Connection 95
Hyperventilation Attack 79, 149, 152, 153, 154, 155
Hyperventilation Syndrome 67, 69, 74, 198
Hyperventilation Test 47
Hypocapnia 70, 113, 130, 133, 151, 167, 179, 193
Hypothyroidism 73, 143, 198

I

IgE 85
Immune system 15, 62, 78, 82, 85, 93, 94, 128, 130, 131, 142, 147,
165, 167, 175, 195
Infection 12, 15, 62, 85, 122, 130, 143, 166, 167, 169, 170, 188,
195, 198, 205, 221, 222, 225
Inflammation 83, 96
Inhalation 90, 96
Inhaled steroids 113
Insomnia 49, 118, 126, 214
Insulin 19, 187, 189, 190, 198
Irritable bowel syndrome 179
Itchy skin 44, 132

K

Keto acid 34
Kidneys 34, 121, 163, 178, 182, 184, 189
Kolb, Peter 216
Kuiper, Dick 218

L

M

N

O

P

Pain 143, 158, 162, 163
Pain Management 158
Panic Attack 9, 41, 67, 149, 150, 151, 152, 156, 229
Parasympathetic nervous system 20, 100, 101
Partial pressure 23, 24, 30
Pavlovich, Konstantin Buteyko 19, 68
pH 2, 17, 18, 20, 21, 22, 23, 30, 32, 34, 52, 105, 109, 120, 121,
133, 145, 151, 178, 179, 188
Physical exercise 66, 81, 136, 137, 143, 154, 160, 179, 195
Pollen 59, 87, 88, 128, 129, 226
Preventer Medication 92
Pulse 53, 76
Pyruvic acid 18, 31

R

Rashes 132
Reduced Breathing 78
Reliever Medication 90
Respiration 25
Respiratory acidosis 22, 38, 105
Respiratory alkalosis 22, 23, 36, 38, 102, 188, 189, 193
Respiratory centre 33, 52, 53, 54, 58, 66, 67, 70, 71, 109, 110, 120
Rhinitis 48, 72, 128, 130
Riddel, Mavis 207

S

Salt 185, 187
Seizure 40, 192, 193, 194
Selye, Hans 11, 144, 197
Semmelweiss, Ignaz 75
Shortness of breath 43, 44, 84, 205
Sighing 44, 228
Sleep Apnoea 118, 123
Sleep apnoea 9, 61, 67, 118, 122, 123, 124, 142, 182, 213
Smooth Muscle 27
Smooth muscle 70, 83, 84, 89, 90, 93, 96, 97, 104, 105, 121, 128,
151, 175, 178, 179, 182
Sneezing 44, 128, 130, 167, 226